Haemorrhage and Thrombosis for the MRCOG and Beyond

Edited by Ann Harper

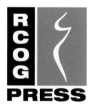

Published by the **RCOG Press**
at the Royal College of Obstetricians and Gynaecologists
27 Sussex Place, Regent's Park, London NW1 4RG

www.rcog.org.uk

Registered charity no. 213280

First published 2005

ISBN 1 900364 96 4

Cover illustration: From Figure 3.1, on page 33.

RCOG Editor: Elisabeth Rees Evans

Index: Cath Topliff

Design/typesetting: Tony Crowley

Printed by Latimer Trend & Co. Ltd., Estover Road, Plymouth PL6 7PL

Contents

About the authors

Rezan Abdul-Kadir MRCOG FRCS(Ed) MD
Consultant Obstetrician and Gynaecologist. Department of Obstetrics and
Gynaecology, Liverpool Road Division, Royal Free Hospital, Pond Street,
London NW3 2QG

Karen Bailie MD PhD MSc(Epid) FRCPath MRCP(UK)
Director, NI Clinical Research Support Centre, Royal Group Hospitals,
Grosvenor Road, Belfast BT12 6BA

Paul Giangrande BSc MD FRCP FRCPath FRCPCH
Consultant Haematologist and Director, Oxford Haemophilia Centre and
Thrombosis Unit, Churchill Hospital, Old Road, Headington, Oxford 0X3 7LJ

Ian Greer MD FRCP(Glas) FRCP(Edin) FRCP(Lond) FRCOG
Regius Professor, Department of Obstetrics and Gynaecology, Glasgow Royal
Infirmary, 10 Alexandra Parade, Glasgow G31 2ER

Ann Harper MD FRCPI FRCOG
Consultant Obstetrician and Gynaecologist, Royal Jubilee Maternity
Service, Grosvenor Road, Belfast BT12 6BA

Pauline Hurley MRCOG
Consultant in Obstetrics and Fetal Medicine, Women's Centre,
The John Radcliffe Hospital, Headley Way, Headington, Oxford 0X3 9DU

Christine Lee MA MD DSc(Med) FRCP FRCPath
Director, Haemophilia Centre and Haemostasis Unit, Royal Free Hospital,
Pond Street, London NW3 2QG

Elizabeth Letsky FRCPath FRCOG FRCPCH
Honorary Consultant Perinatal Haematologist, Queen Charlotte's and
Chelsea Hospital, Du Cane Road, London W12 0HS

Michael F Murphy MD FRCPath
Consultant Haematologist, National Blood Service, Department of Haematology,
Oxford Radcliffe Hospitals & University of Oxford, Headley Way, Headington,
Oxford OX3 9DU

Jane E Ramsay MD MRCOG
Clinical Lecturer, Department of Obsterics and Gynaecology, University of
Glasgow, Glasgow Royal Infirmary, Macewen Building, Glasgow G4 0SF

Isobel Walker MD FRCP(Ed) FRCPath
Consultant Haematologist, Department of Haematology,
Glasgow Royal Infirmary, 3rd Floor, Macewen Building, Glasgow G4 0SF

Abbreviations

ADP	adenosine diphosphate
aPC	activated protein C
aPL	antiphospholipid antibodies
APTT	activated partial thromboplastin time
AT	antithrombin
βhCG	beta human chorionic gonadotrophin
BMI	body mass index
CEMD	Confidential Enquiries into Maternal Deaths
CT	computed tomography
DDAVP	1-desamino-8-D-arginine vasopressin
DIC	disseminated intravascular coagulation
DVT	deep vein thrombosis
ESR	erythrocyte sedimentation rate
FBS	fetal blood sampling
FDP	fibrin degradation product
FVL	factor V Leiden
HELLP	haemolysis, elevated liver enzymes and low platelet count
HLA	human leucocyte antigen
HPA	human platelet antigens
HRT	hormone replacement therapy
INR	international normalised ratio
ITP	idiopathic thrombocytopenic purpura
IVIgG	intravenous immunoglobulin G
LMWH	low molecular weight heparin
MRI	magnetic resonance imaging
NAIT	neonatal alloimmune thrombocytopenia
OCP	combined oral contraceptives
PBAC	pictorial blood assessment chart
PC	protein C
PS	protein S
PT	prothrombin time
PTE	pulmonary embolism

TORCH	toxoplasmosis, other (congenital syphilis and viruses), rubella, cytomegalovirus and herpes simplex virus
TT	thrombin time
UFH	unfractionated heparin
V/Q	ventilation/perfusion
VTE	venous thromboembolism
VWD	von Willebrand's disorder
VWF	von Willebrand factor

Preface

Although disorders of the coagulation system are uncommon in pregnancy, the two main hazards, haemorrhage and thromboembolism, are leading causes of direct maternal death in the UK and worldwide. The fetus may be seriously affected by some bleeding disorders and by the consequences of major maternal haemorrhage or thromboembolism. Gynaecologists may encounter abnormal haemostasis as a cause of intractable menorrhagia or perioperative haemorrhage, and thromboembolism is a significant risk for women undergoing major gynaecological surgery. As more is discovered about the coagulation system, it is becoming apparent that some women are at increased risk of haemorrhage or thrombosis. This book, which brings together various aspects of haemostasis in relation to obstetrics and gynaecology, will be useful to candidates preparing for the MRCOG examination and may provide some practical guidance for doctors who only occasionally encounter these conditions. Good working relationships and close liaison between obstetricians and gynaecologists, anaesthetists, haematologists, and the blood transfusion service are essential to ensure the best outcome for women with disturbances of haemostasis or thrombosis. My appreciation and thanks to all the contributors.

Ann Harper

1 The coagulation system in pregnancy

During pregnancy, major changes occur in the components of the coagulation system. Some of these physiological adaptations are unique to human pregnancy. Their significance and their relation to haemorrhage and thrombosis, which are major hazards for the pregnant woman, can only be appreciated with knowledge of the haemostatic mechanisms in the healthy nonpregnant individual.

The integrity and patency of the vascular tree is dependent on a finely controlled interaction between the coagulation system and fibrinolysis.

To make the pathology and management of haemostatic disorders more understandable, a short account of haemostasis during pregnancy and how it differs from that in the nonpregnant state follows.

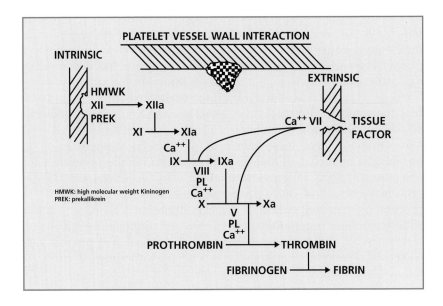

Figure 1.1 The interacting haemostatic/coagulation pathways

Haemostasis and pregnancy

Healthy haemostasis depends upon normal vasculature, platelets, coagulation factors and fibrinolysis. These act together to confine the circulating blood to the vascular bed, maintain its fluidity and arrest bleeding after trauma (Figure 1.1). Normal pregnancy is accompanied by dramatic changes in the coagulation and fibrinolytic systems, with a marked increase in some of the procoagulant factors, particularly fibrinogen, and suppression of fibrinolysis.[1–3] These changes, together with a significant increase in total blood volume, help to combat the hazard of haemorrhage at placental separation but play only a secondary role to the unique process of myometrial contraction, which reduces blood flow to the placental site. They also produce a vulnerable state for intravascular clotting, which is expressed as a whole spectrum of disorders ranging from thromboembolism to haemorrhage resulting from disseminated intravascular coagulation (DIC).[4]

Vascular integrity

It is not known how vascular integrity is normally maintained but it is clear that the platelets have a key role, since conditions in which their number is depleted or their function is abnormal are characterised by widespread spontaneous capillary haemorrhages. It is thought that the platelets in health are constantly sealing microdefects of the vasculature by forming miniature fibrin clots, the unwanted fibrin being removed by fibrinolysis. Generation of prostacyclin appears to be the physiological mechanism which protects the vessel wall from excess deposition of platelet aggregates, and explains why contact of platelets with healthy vascular endothelium is not a stimulus for thrombus formation.[5]

Prostacyclin (PGI_2) is an unstable prostaglandin first discovered in 1976. It is the principal prostanoid that blood vessels synthesise, a powerful vasodilator and a potent inhibitor of platelet aggregation. Moncada and Vane[5] proposed that there is a balance between the production of prostacyclin by the vessel wall, and the production of the vasoconstrictor and powerful aggregating agent thromboxane by the platelet. Prostacyclin prevents adhesion at much lower concentrations than are needed to prevent aggregation; vascular damage, therefore, leads to platelet adhesion but not necessarily to aggregation and thrombus formation.

Prostacyclin synthetase is abundant in the intima and progressively decreases in concentration from the subendothelium to the adventitia. It follows that severe vessel damage or physical detachment of the endothelium will lead to the development of a large thrombus as opposed to simple platelet adherence.

There are several conditions in which the production of prostacyclin could be impaired, thereby upsetting the normal balance. Prostacyclin production has been shown to be reduced in fetal and placental tissue from pre-eclamptic pregnancies, and the current role of prostacyclin in the pathogenesis of pre-eclampsia continues to undergo investigation.

The endothelium is now regarded as an extremely important component of the haemostatic system; endothelial cell injury leads to platelet activation and triggering of the coagulation system. It is possible that the changes in haemostatic components are purely a secondary response to underlying vascular disease.

Some studies have shown an increased oxygen free radical production in pre-eclampsia, which will in turn decrease vascular prostacyclin and endothelial-dependent relaxing factor (i.e. nitric oxide), and release and increase thromboxane A_2. The whole subject of endothelial function in pre-eclampsia has been well reviewed.[6]

Platelets

Platelets are produced in the bone marrow by the megakaryocytes and have a lifespan of 9–12 days. At the end of their normal lifespan the effete cells are engulfed by cells of the reticulo-endothelial system and most damaged platelets are sequestered in the spleen.

There have been conflicting reports concerning the platelet count during normal pregnancy. A review of publications over 25 years[7] revealed a majority consensus (of six), suggesting a small fall in the platelet count towards term, during normal pregnancy. However, few of these studies obtained longitudinal data and none performed a within-patient analysis. Now that automated platelet counting is routine as part of the full blood count, more information is available about the platelet count in normal, uncomplicated pregnancy. It is becoming clear that, if mean values for platelet concentration are analysed throughout pregnancy, there is a downward trend[8] even though the majority fall within the accepted nonpregnant range.[7,9,10]

There is also conflicting evidence[11,12] of increased platelet turnover and low grade platelet activation as pregnancy advances, resulting in a larger proportion of younger platelets with a greater mean platelet volume.[7,8]

Most investigators agree that low-grade chronic intravascular coagulation within the uteroplacental circulation is a part of the physiological response of all women to pregnancy. This is partially compensated and it is not surprising that the platelets should be involved either giving indices of increased turnover or in some cases a reduction in number.

A prospective study of 2263 healthy women delivering during one year at a Canadian obstetric centre[13] showed that 8.3% had mild thrombocytopenia at term (platelet counts 97–150 x 10^9/l). The frequency of thrombocytopenia in their offspring was no greater than that of babies born to women with platelet counts in the normal accepted range and no infant had a platelet count <100 x 10^9/l. An extension of this study to include 6715 deliveries substantiates these original findings.[14]

In one study, women with a normal pregnancy were compared with nonpregnant controls. They were shown to have a significantly lower platelet count and an increase in circulating platelet aggregates. *In vitro* the platelets were shown to be hypoaggregable. This was interpreted as suggesting platelet activation during pregnancy causing platelet aggregation and followed by exhaustion of platelets.[15]

Earlier publications suggesting that there was no evidence of changes in platelet function or differences in platelet lifespan[11,16] between healthy nonpregnant and pregnant women have to be re-evaluated in the face of more recent investigations, but it is clear that normal pregnancy has little significant effect on the screening parameter that is usually measured, namely the platelet count.

The problem remains in defining completely normal pregnancy. Certain disease states specific to pregnancy have profound effects on platelet consumption, lifespan and function.

Platelets in pre-eclampsia

A decrease in platelet count[17] and changes in platelet function[18] have been observed in pregnancies with fetal growth restriction and the lifespan of platelets is shortened significantly even in mild pre-eclampsia.[19,20]

Many reports and reviews have shown that the circulating platelet count is reduced in pre-eclampsia.[21,22] A fall in the platelet count may precede any detectable rise in serum fibrin degradation products (FDP) in women subsequently developing pre-eclampsia. The platelet count can be used to monitor severity of the disease process as well as for initial screening if there is concern about significant coagulation abnormalities.[23]

Thrombocytopenia

The most common platelet abnormality encountered in clinical practice is thrombocytopenia. During the hundred years since platelets were first described an increasing understanding of their role in haemostasis and thrombosis has taken place. At the same time there have been dramatic reductions in maternal and fetal mortality, but maternal thrombocytopenia remains a difficult management problem during pregnancy and can also have profound effects on fetal and neonatal wellbeing.

A low platelet count is seen most frequently in association with DIC whether it is low grade, uncompensated or rampant with haemorrhage (Table 1.1; see Chapter 5).

Table 1.1 Spectrum of severity of disseminated intravascular coagulation (DIC): its relationship to specific complications in obstetrics

Stage	Severity of DIC	In vitro findings	Commonly associated obstetric conditions
1	Low-grade compensated	FDPs ↑ Increased soluble fibrin complexes Increased ratio vWFa/factor VIIIC	Pre-eclampsia Retained dead fetus
2	Uncompensated but no haemostatic failure	As above, plus fibrinogen ↓ Platelets ↓	Small placental abruption Severe pre-eclampsia
3	Rampant with haemostatic failure	Platelets ↓↓ Gross depletion of coagulation factors, particularly fibrinogen FDPs ↑↑	Placental abruption Amniotic fluid embolism Eclampsia

FDPs = fibrin degradation products; vWF = von Willebrand factor

Probably the single most important cause of isolated thrombocytopenia is autoimmune idiopathic thrombocytopenic purpura (ITP), which is a disease primarily of young women in the reproductive years.[24]

The causes and management of maternal and fetal thrombocytopenia have been reviewed[25–27] and are dealt with in Chapter 3.

Arrest of bleeding after trauma

An essential function of the haemostatic system is a rapid reaction to injury which remains confined to the area of damage. This requires a control mechanism which will stimulate coagulation after trauma, and also limit the extent of the response. The substances involved in the formation of the haemostatic plug normally circulate in an inert form, until activated at the site of injury, or by some other factor released into the circulation which will trigger intravascular coagulation (Figure 1.2).

Local response

Platelets adhere to collagen on the injured basement membrane, which triggers a series of changes in the platelets themselves, including shape change and release of adenosine diphosphate (ADP) and other substances.

Release of ADP stimulates further aggregation of platelets, which triggers the coagulation cascade generating thrombin; this in turn leads to the formation of fibrin which converts the platelet plug into a firm, stable wound seal. The role of platelets is of less importance in injury involving large vessels, because platelet aggregates are of insufficient size and strength to close the defect. The coagulation mechanism is of major importance here, together with vascular contraction.

Coagulation system

The end result of blood coagulation is the formation of an insoluble fibrin clot from the soluble precursor fibrinogen in the plasma. This involves a complex interaction of clotting factors, and a sequential activation of a

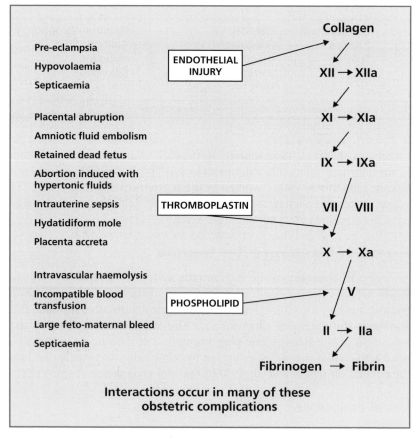

Figure 1.2 Trigger mechanisms of disseminated intravascular coagulation during pregnancy

series of pro-enzymes, the coagulation cascade (Figure 1.3). When a blood vessel is injured, blood coagulation is initiated by activation of factor XII by collagen (intrinsic mechanism) and activation of factor VII by thromboplastin release (extrinsic mechanism) from the damaged tissues. Both the intrinsic and extrinsic mechanisms are activated by components of the vessel wall and both are required for normal haemostasis. Strict divisions between the two pathways do not exist and interactions between activated factors in both pathways have been shown. They share a common pathway following the activation of factor X (Figures 1.1 and 1.3).

The intrinsic pathway (or contact system) proceeds spontaneously and is relatively slow, requiring 5–20 minutes for visible fibrin formation. All tissues contain a specific lipoprotein, thromboplastin (particularly concentrated in lung and brain), which markedly increases the rate at which blood clots. The placenta is also rich in tissue factor (thromboplastin), which will produce fibrin formation within 12 seconds; the acceleration of coagulation is brought about by bypassing the reactions involving the contact (intrinsic) system (Figure 1.3). Since blood coagulation is strictly confined to the site of tissue injury in normal circumstances, powerful control mechanisms must be at work to prevent

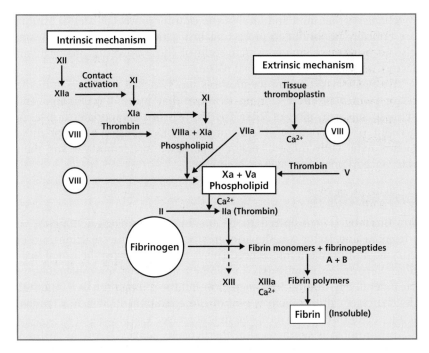

Figure 1.3 The factors involved in blood coagulation and their interactions

dissemination of coagulation.

Normal pregnancy is accompanied by major changes in the coagulation system, with increases in levels of factors VII, VIII and X, and a particularly marked increase in the level of plasma fibrinogen[28] (Figure 1.3), which is probably the chief cause of the accelerated erythrocyte sedimentation rate (ESR) observed during normal pregnancy. In the second half of pregnancy, the 95th centile for ESR was shown to be 70 mm/hour in a large group of healthy women studied at Queen Charlotte's Hospital, London.[29] The effect of pregnancy on the coagulation factors can be detected from about the third month of gestation, and the amount of fibrinogen in late pregnancy is at least double that of the nonpregnant state.[28]

However, the single most important component of haemostasis at delivery is contraction of the myometrium stemming the flow from the placental site. Massive transfusion of all clotting factors and platelets will not stop haemorrhage if the uterus remains flabby. Vaginal delivery will make less severe demand on the haemostatic mechanism than delivery by caesarean section, which requires the same haemostatic competence as any other major surgical procedure.

The naturally occurring anticoagulants

Mechanisms that limit and localise the clotting process at sites of trauma are critically important to protect against generalised thrombosis – and also to prevent spontaneous activation of those powerful procoagulant factors which circulate in normal plasma.

Investigation of healthy haemostasis has switched emphasis from the factors which promote clotting to those that prevent generalised and spontaneous activation of these factors. It is not appropriate to give an account of the complex interactions and biochemistry of all of these factors here. Only those of major importance in haemostasis and their relevance to pregnancy will be mentioned.

Antithrombin

Antithrombin is considered to be the main physiological inhibitor of thrombin and factor Xa. Heparin greatly enhances the reaction rate of enzyme antithrombin interaction. This is the rationale for the use of low-dose heparin as prophylaxis in women at risk of thromboembolism postoperatively, and during pregnancy and the puerperium. An inherited deficiency of antithrombin is one of the conditions in which a familial tendency to thrombosis has been described (see Chapter 8).

Antithrombin is synthesised in the liver. Its activity is low in cirrhosis and other chronic diseases of the liver, as well as in protein-losing renal disease, DIC and hypercoagulable states. The most common cause of a small reduction in antithrombin is the use of oral contraceptives; this effect is related to the oestrogen content of the pill.

During healthy pregnancy there is little change in antithrombin level but there is some decrease at parturition and an increase in the puerperium.[28] However, there must be increased synthesis in the antenatal period to maintain normal concentrations in the face of an increasing plasma volume.

Protein C-thrombomodulin-protein S

Protein C inactivates factors V and VIII in conjunction with its cofactors thrombomodulin and protein S. Protein C is a vitamin K-dependent anticoagulant synthesised in the liver. To exert its effect it must be activated by an endothelial cell cofactor termed thrombomodulin. The importance of the protein C-thrombomodulin-protein S system is exemplified by the absence of thrombomodulin in the brain where the priority for haemostasis is higher than for anticoagulation.

Many kindreds with a deficiency or a functional deficit of protein C with associated recurrent thromboembolism have been described[30] (see Chapter 8). Purpura fulminans neonatalis is the homozygous expression of protein C deficiency with severe thrombosis and neonatal death.[31]

Protein S, also a vitamin K-dependent glycoprotein, acts as a cofactor for activated protein C by promoting its binding to lipid and platelet surface thus localising the reaction.

Many families have been reported with protein S deficiency and thromboembolic disease.

Data on protein C and protein S levels in healthy pregnancy are sparse. One study showed a significant reduction in functional protein S levels during pregnancy and the puerperium.[32] Fourteen women followed longitudinally throughout gestation and postpartum showed a rise of protein C within the normal nonpregnant range during the second trimester. In contrast free protein S fell from the second trimester onwards but remained within the confines of the normal range.[33]

Another study supported these findings and extended them to include women using oral contraceptives in whom similar changes were found.[34]

Although the investigation of natural anticoagulants has only just begun, the system has grown in complexity as our knowledge has increased. There is little doubt that in the future more components will be recognised as our ability to investigate objectively increases,[35] allowing a better and more thorough understanding of the mechanisms underlying the control of the delicate balance between procoagulant and anticoagulant factors[36] and enabling us to manage these complex hypercoagulable states in pregnancy successfully.[37]

Activated protein C resistance

Activated protein C (aPC) resistance is a familial thrombophilic tendency characterised by poor anticoagulant response to activated protein C, caused in the vast majority of cases by a single mutation in the factor V gene – factor V Leiden.[38] Investigations in normal pregnancy have shown an increasing resistance to activated protein C with gestation.[39–41] One explanation for the increased aPC resistance could be the significant rise in factor VIII procoagulant activity which accompanies healthy pregnancy. At least one study found a correlation between rising factor VIII activity and increased aPC resistance.[41]

Pathological thrombophilia

The roles of antithrombin, protein C and S deficiency, factor V Leiden and the prothrombin gene variant together with other genetic and acquired thrombophilia factors in pregnancy are discussed in Chapter 8.[42,43]

Fibrinolysis

Fibrinolytic activity is an essential part of the dynamic, interacting haemostatic mechanism, and is dependent upon plasminogen activator in the blood (Figure 1.4). Fibrin and fibrinogen are digested by plasmin, a pro-enzyme derived from an inactive plasma precursor plasminogen.

Increased amounts of activator are found in the plasma after strenuous exercise, emotional stress, surgical operations and other trauma. Tissue activator can be extracted from most human organs with the exception of the placenta. Tissues especially rich in activator include the uterus, ovaries, prostate, heart, lungs, thyroid, adrenals and lymph nodes. Activity in tissues is concentrated mainly around blood vessels, veins showing greater activity than arteries.

The inhibitors of fibrinolytic activity are of two types – anti-activator (antiplasminogens) and the antiplasmins. Inhibitors of plasminogen include epsilon amino caproic acid and tranexamic acid. Aprotinin (Trasylol®) is another antiplasminogen which is commercially prepared from bovine lung.

Platelets, plasma and serum exert a strong inhibitory action on plasmin. Normally, plasma antiplasmin levels exceed levels of plasminogen and hence the levels of potential plasmin; otherwise we would dissolve away our connecting cement! When fibrinogen or fibrin is broken down by plasmin, fibrin degradation products are formed; these comprise the high molecular weight split products X and Y, and smaller fragments, A, B, C, D and E (Figure 1.5). When a fibrin clot is formed, 70% of fragment X is retained in the clot, Y, D and E being retained to a somewhat lesser extent. Note that blood for estimation of FDPs should be taken by clean venepuncture. The

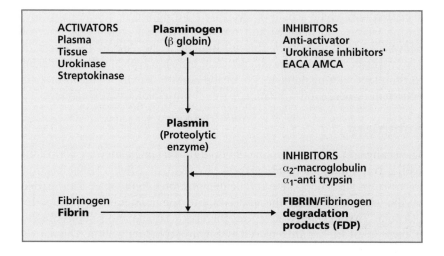

Figure 1.4 Components of the fibrinolytic system

tourniquet should not be left on too long since venous stasis also stimulates fibrinolytic activity. The blood should be allowed to clot in the presence of an antifibrinolytic agent such as epsilon amino caproic acid to stop the process of fibrinolysis, which would otherwise continue *in vitro*.

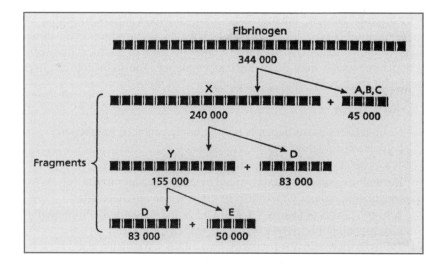

Figure 1.5 Fibrin degradation products produced by action of plasma fibrinogen; the molecular weights are shown

Plasma fibrinolytic activity is decreased during pregnancy, remains low during labour and delivery and returns to normal within one hour of delivery of the placenta.[44] This is thought to be due to the effect of placentally derived plasminogen activator inhibitor type 2, which is present in abundance during pregnancy.[45] In addition the activity in the fibrinolytic system in response to stimulation is significantly reduced in pregnancy.[46]

Summary

The changes in the coagulation system in normal pregnancy are consistent with a continuing low grade process of coagulant activity. Using electron microscopy, fibrin deposition can be demonstrated in the intervillous space of the placenta and in the walls of the spiral arteries supplying the placenta.[47] As pregnancy advances, the elastic lamina and smooth muscle of these spiral arteries are replaced by a matrix containing fibrin. This allows expansion of the lumen to accommodate an increasing blood flow and reduces the vascular resistance of the placenta. At placental separation during normal childbirth, a blood flow of 500–800 ml/min has to be staunched within seconds, or serious haemorrhage will occur. Myometrial contraction plays a vital role in securing haemostasis by reducing the blood flow to the placental site. Rapid closure of the terminal part of the spiral artery will be further facilitated by removal of the elastic lamina. The placental site is rapidly covered by a fibrin mesh following delivery. The increased levels of fibrinogen and other coagulation factors will be advantageous to meet the sudden demand for haemostatic components but, around delivery, haemorrhage still remains a significant cause of maternal morbidity and mortality.[48] The changes also produce a vulnerable state for intravascular clotting and a whole spectrum of disorders involving coagulation which may occur during pregnancy. The following chapters deal with the investigation and management of these disorders.

Key points

1 Normal haemostasis depends upon a finely balanced interaction between coagulation and fibrinolysis.

2 The platelet count falls in normal pregnancy.

3 Normal pregnancy is accompanied by major changes in the coagulation system which help to prevent haemorrhage after delivery. Levels of factors VII, VIII and X and particularly fibrinogen increase while fibrinolytic activity is decreased.

4 These changes convert prenancy into a hypercoagulable state, increasing the risk of thromboembolism.

5 Myometrial contraction following separation of the placenta is the main mechanism which prevents serious haemorrhage.

References

1   Stirling Y, Woolf L, North WR, et al. Haemostasis in normal pregnancy. *Thromb Haemost* 1984;52(2):176–82.

2   Forbes CD, Greer IA. Physiology of haemostasis and the effect of pregnancy. In: Forbes CD, Greer IA, editors. *Haemostasis and Thrombosis in Obstetrics and Gynaecology*. London: Chapman & Hall; 1992. p. 1–25.

3   Letsky EA. Mechanisms of coagulation and the changes induced by pregnancy. *Curr Obstet Gynaecol* 1991;1:203–9.

4   Levi M,Ten Cate H. Disseminated Intravascular Coagulation. *N Engl J Med* 1999;341(8):586–92.

5   Moncada S, Vane JR. Arachidonic acid metabolites and the interactions between platelets and blood-vessel walls. *N Engl J Med* 1979;300(20):1142–7.

6   Zeeman GG, Dekker GA, van Geijn HP, *et al.* Endothelial function in normal and pre-eclamptic pregnancy: a hypothesis. *Eur J Obstet Gynecol Reprod Biol* 1992;43(2):113–22.

7   Sill PR, Lind T, Walker W. Platelet values during normal pregnancy. *Br J Obstet Gynaecol* 1985;92(5):480–83.

8   Fay RA, Hughes AO, Farron NT. Platelets in pregnancy: hyperdestruction in pregnancy. *Obstet Gynecol* 1983;61(2):238–40.

9   Beal DW, De Masi AD. Role of the platelet count in management of the high-risk obstetric patient. *J Am Osteopath Assoc* 1985;85(4):252–5.

10 Fenton V, Saunders K, Cavill I. The platelet count in pregnancy. *J Clin Path* 1977;30(1):68–9.

11 Rakoczi I, Tallian F, Bagdany S, *et al.* Platelet life-span in normal pregnancy and pre-eclampsia as determined by a non-radioisotope technique. *Thromb Res* 1979;15(3–4):553-56.

12 Wallenburg HC, van Kessel PH. Platelet lifespan in normal pregnancy as determined by a nonradioisotopic technique. *Br J Obstet Gynaecol* 1978;85(1):33–6.

13 Burrows RF, Kelton JG. Incidentally detected thrombocytopenia in healthy mothers and their infants. *N Engl J Med* 1988;319(3):142–5.

14 Burrows RF, Kelton JG. Thrombocytopenia at delivery: a prospective survey of 6715 deliveries. *Am J Obstet Gynecol* 1990;162(3):731–4.

15 O'Brien WF, Saba HI, Knuppel RA, *et al.* Alterations in platelet concentration and aggregation in normal pregnancy and preeclampsia. *Am J Obstet Gynecol* 1986;155(3):486–90.

16 Romero R, Duffy TP. Platelet disorders in pregnancy. *Clin Perinatol* 1980;7(2):327–48.

17 Redman CW, Bonnar J, Beilin L. Early platelet consumption in pre-eclampsia. *Br Med J* 1978;1(6111):467–9.

18 Ahmed Y, Sullivan MH, Pearce JM, *et al.* Changes in platelet function in pregnancies complicated by fetal growth retardation. *Eur J Obstet Gynecol Reprod Biol* 1991;42(3):171–5.

19 Ballegeer VC, Spitz B, De Baene LA, *et al.* Platelet activation and vascular damage in gestational hypertension. *Am J Obstet Gynecol* 1992;166(2):629–33.

20 Lin KC, Chou TC, Yin CS, *et al*. The role of aggregation of platelets in pregnancy-induced hypertension: a comprehensive and longitudinal study. *Int J Cardiol* 1991;33(1):125–31.

21 Baker P, Cunningham F. Platelet and Coagulation Abnormalities. In: Baker P, Cunningham F, editors. *Chesley's Hypertensive Disorders in Pregnancy*. Stamford, Conn: Appleton & Lange; 1999. p. 349–73.

22 Romero R, Mazor M, Lockwood CJ, *et al*. Clinical significance, prevalence, and natural history of thrombocytopenia in pregnancy-induced hypertension. *Am J Perinatol* 1989;6(1):32–8.

23 Leduc L, Wheeler JM, Kirshon B, *et al*. Coagulation profile in severe preeclampsia. *Obstet Gynecol* 1992;79(1):14–18.

24 McMillan R. Chronic idiopathic thrombocytopenic purpura. *N Engl J Med* 1981;304:1135–7.

25 Colvin BT. Thrombocytopenia. In: Colvin BT, editor. *Haematological Disorders in Pregnancy*. London: WB Saunders; 1985. p. 661–81.

26 Pillai M. Platelets and pregnancy. *Br J Obstet Gynaecol* 1993;100:201–4.

27 Letsky EA, Greaves M. Guidelines on the investigation and management of thrombocytopenia in pregnancy and neonatal alloimmune thrombocytopenia. *Br J Haematol* 1996;95:21–6.

28 Hellgren M, Blomback M. Studies on blood coagulation and fibrinolysis in pregnancy, during delivery and in the puerperium. I. Normal condition. *Gyneco Obstet Invest* 1981;12(3):141–54.

29 Van den Broek N, Letsky E. Pregnancy and the erythrocyte sedimentation rate. *Br J Obstet Gynaecol* 2001;108:1164–7.

30 Bertina RM, Briet E, Engesser L, *et al*. Protein C deficiency and the risk of venous thrombosis. *N Engl J Med* 1988;318:930–31.

31 Seligsohn U, Berger A, Abend M, *et al*. Homozygous protein C deficiency manifested by massive venous thrombosis in the newborn. *N Engl J Med* 1984;310(9):559–62.

32 Comp PC, Thurnau GR, Welsh J, *et al*. Functional and immunologic protein S levels are decreased during pregnancy. *Blood* 1986;68(4):881–5.

33 Warwick R, Hutton RA, Goff L, *et al*. Changes in protein C and free protein S during pregnancy and following hysterectomy. *J R Soc Med* 1989;82(10):591–4.

34 Malm J, Laurell M, Dahlback B. Changes in the plasma levels of vitamin K-dependent proteins C and S and of C4b-binding protein during pregnancy and oral contraception. *Br J Haematol* 1988;68(4):437–43.

35 Alving BM, Comp PC. Recent advances in understanding clotting and evaluating patients with recurrent thrombosis. *Am J Obstet Gynecol* 1992; 167(4Pt2):1184–91.

36 Salem HH. The natural anticoagulants. In: Salem HH, editor. *Thrombosis and the Vessel Wall, Clinics in Haematology*. London: WB Saunders; 1986. p. 371–91.

37 Walker ID. Management of thrombophilia in pregnancy. *Blood Rev* 1991; 5(4):227–33.

38 Bertina RM, Koeleman RPC, Koster T, *et al*. Mutation in blood coagulation factor V associated with resistance to activated protein C. *Nature* 1994;369:64–7.

39 Hellgren M, Svensson PJ, Dahlback B. Resistance to activated protein C as a basis for venous thromboembolism associated with pregnancy and oral contraceptives. *Am J Obstet Gynecol* 1995;173(1):210–13.

40 Cumming AM, Tait RC, Fildes S, *et al.* Development of resistance to activated protein C during pregnancy. *Br J Haematol* 1995;90:725–7.

41 Peek MJ, Nelson-Piercy C, Manning RA, *et al.* Activated protein C resistance in normal pregnancy. *Br J Obstet Gynaecol* 1997;104:1084–6.

42 Kupferminc MJ, Eldor A, Steinman N, *et al.* Increased Frequency of Genetic Thrombophilia in Women with Complications of Pregnancy. *N Engl J Med* 1999;340:9–13.

43 Haemostasis and Thrombosis Task Force and British Committee for Standards in Haematology. Guideline: Investigation and management of heritable thrombophilia. *Br J Haematol* 2001;114:512–28.

44 Bonnar J, Prentice CRM, McNicol GP, *et al.* Haemostatic mechanism in uterine circulation during placental separation. *Br Med J* 1971;2:564–7.

45 Booth NA, Reith A, Bennett B. A plasminogen activator inhibitor (PAI-2) circulates in two molecular forms during pregnancy. *Thromb Haemost* 1988;59(1):77–9.

46 Ballegeer V, Mombaerts P, Declerck PJ, *et al.* Fibrinolytic response to venous occlusion and fibrin fragment D-dimer levels in normal and complicated pregnancy. *Thromb Haemost* 1987;58(4):1030–32.

47 Sheppard BL, Bonnar J. The ultrastructure of the arterial supply of the human placenta in early and late pregnancy. *J Obstet Gynaecol Br Commonw* 1974;81(7):497–511.

48 Hall MH. Haemorrhage. In: Lewis G, Drife J, editors. *Why Mothers Die 2000–2002. The Sixth Report of the Confidential Enquiries into Maternal Deaths in the United Kingdom.* London: RCOG Press; 2004. p. 86–95.

2 Pregnancy in women with inherited bleeding disorders

This chapter deals with the management of pregnancy and delivery in women who suffer from, or are carriers of, an inherited bleeding disorder such as von Willebrand's disease or haemophilia, or are female partners of affected men. These women should have prepregnancy counselling, including genetic counselling. If there is a possibility that they may require treatment with blood products and they are not already immune, they should also be immunised against hepatitis A and B. Pregnancy and delivery should be managed with close liaison between the obstetric and haematology teams, preferably allied with a haemophilia centre. Good communication and written protocols are important. Delivery should be in a maternity unit with ready access to blood and blood products and neonatal intensive care facilities.

Haemophilia

Haemophilia A is a congenital disorder of coagulation, characterised by deficiency of factor VIII in the blood. Deficiency of factor IX results in an identical clinical condition known as haemophilia B (also known as Christmas disease). Haemophilia is encountered in all racial groups, with an incidence of approximately one in 10 000. The clinical picture is dependent upon the degree of deficiency of the coagulation factor in the blood: severe haemophilia is associated with a level of less than 1% of normal. The hallmark of severe haemophilia is recurrent and spontaneous bleeding into joints, principally the knees, elbows and ankles. Repeated bleeding into joints can, in the absence of treatment, result in disabling arthritis at an early age. Bleeding into muscles and soft tissues is also seen frequently. Advances in the treatment of haemophilia have led to improvements in both longevity and quality of life of people with even severe haemophilia. As these people live longer and integrate fully into society, it is expected that the numbers of people with severe haemophilia will increase significantly because the daughters of haemophiliacs are obligate carriers of the condition. Obstetricians will thus be faced more frequently with the problem of management of pregnancy in known or possible carriers of this condition.

CARRIERS OF HAEMOPHILIA

The genes for both factor VIII and IX are located on the X chromosome and thus inheritance is sex-linked and recessive, like colour blindness. The daughters of men with haemophilia are obligate carriers, with a 50:50 chance of passing on the condition to a son and a similar chance that a daughter will be a carrier of the condition (Figure 2.1). Homozygous haemophilia A or B in women may occur rarely (e.g. in females who are the offspring of a haemophiliac father and a carrier mother) and these women are affected in the same way as haemophilic males.

The severity of haemophilia within a given family remains constant. If a woman has relatives with only mild haemophilia, she may be reassured that there is no risk of transmitting a severe form of the disease. However, one-third of cases arise in families with no previous family history, and reflect new mutations. The most famous example of this phenomenon was the British Queen, Victoria (1819–1901), who gave birth to a haemophilic son, Leopold, in 1853.

Most female carriers of haemophilia have levels of factor VIII (or IX) within the normal range but a significant proportion will have a modest reduction in the baseline level. The baseline level is seldom lower than 20% of the normal level and should suffice to protect against significant bleeding problems in day-to-day life. However, female carriers with low levels of factor VIII (or IX) are at risk of bleeding during surgery or other invasive procedures such as dental extractions or biopsies. In such circumstances, haemostatic support may be required and the choice of

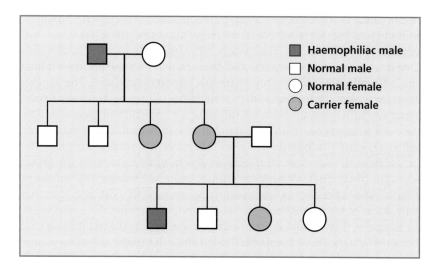

Figure 2.1 The sex-linked recessive inheritance of haemophilia

product will depend on both the factor level and the nature of the procedure. Recombinant coagulation factor concentrates should be considered to be the products of choice in such cases.

There is no need to carry out genetic tests to determine the carrier status of the daughters of men with haemophilia because they are obligate carriers. However, genotypic analysis to determine the underlying genetic defect should be offered as this will facilitate antenatal testing (see below) in due course, if required. The carrier status for other women in an extended family may not be so clear: a woman who has an affected uncle, for example, may or may not be a carrier. An all too common and difficult problem is to be confronted with a pregnant woman with a vague history of a bleeding disorder in a distant relative. Carrier testing can take some months to perform and it may therefore seem logical to determine carrier status as soon as possible in girls with a family history of the condition, as this would facilitate management in an early and unexpected pregnancy. However, testing of young children ignores the ethical and legal rights of children as the informed consent of the individual child concerned cannot be considered to have been obtained. These issues must be discussed openly with the family. Once the carrier status has been determined and the specific genetic defect has been identified, it is then possible to offer antenatal diagnosis of haemophilia to pregnant women.

ANTENATAL DIAGNOSIS OF HAEMOPHILIA

Social and cultural attitudes to termination of pregnancy vary considerably around the world. As a general rule, antenatal diagnosis of haemophilia is offered only where termination of the pregnancy would be contemplated if an affected fetus were identified. It is certainly not necessary to determine the status of a male fetus simply to plan management of the pregnancy and delivery. Women require counselling about haemophilia before they make this important decision. The general experience has been that only a minority of women in developed countries subsequently take up the offer of antenatal diagnosis with a view to termination if an affected fetus is identified.[1,2] This may well reflect the fact that many women with affected relatives recognise the tremendous advances in treatment in recent years, including the wider adoption of prophylaxis and the introduction of recombinant products, which have resulted in an essentially normal life for the younger generation of haemophiliacs.

Chorionic villus sampling, or biopsy, is the principal method used for antenatal diagnosis of haemophilia. It offers the major advantage over amniocentesis of permitting diagnosis during the first trimester, although it should not be carried out before 11 weeks of gestation because earlier biopsy may be associated with a risk of subsequent fetal limb abnormalities.[3,4] The sample of chorionic villus is obtained by either the transabdominal or transvaginal route, under ultrasound guidance, and is then subjected to DNA analysis. It is possible that in the not too distant future noninvasive antenatal diagnostic procedures may become available in which fetal DNA can be extracted from fetal normoblasts in the maternal circulation.[5]

Fetal blood sampling is carried out when it has not been possible to establish the status of the fetus through DNA-based tests. In this technique, fetal blood is taken from fetal umbilical vessels under ultrasound guidance at around 15–19 weeks of gestation. Approximately 1 ml of blood is required for assay of coagulation factor levels. The levels of factor VIII and IX in a normal fetus at around 19 weeks of gestation are significantly lower than in an adult, at approximately 40 iu/dl and 10 iu/dl respectively.[6,7] It is therefore essential to ensure that the blood is wholly fetal and not contaminated with maternal blood, which could result in diagnostic error through spurious elevation of the factor level in the sample. This may be done rapidly (during the procedure) by measuring the mean corpuscular volume of the erythrocytes with a red cell counter. The fetal mean corpuscular volume is typically at least 120 fl at this stage of pregnancy, while that of the mother is around 90 fl. The Kleihauer technique, based on demonstrating resistance of fetal haemoglobin to acid elution, is more reliable but takes longer to carry out. The factor assay results should never be communicated without results of such additional tests to confirm the fetal origin of the sample.

All invasive methods used for antenatal diagnosis may cause feto-maternal haemorrhage, and anti-D immunoglobulin should be given in the usual fashion if the mother is rhesus D negative. These procedures are likely to be carried out early in pregnancy, when the factor VIII level has not risen significantly, and so it is quite possible that some form of haemostatic support may be required to prevent maternal bleeding.

MANAGEMENT OF DELIVERY IN CARRIERS OF HAEMOPHILIA

The levels of factor VIII and von Willebrand factor (VWF) rise during normal pregnancy (Figure 2.2). The rise is particularly marked during the third trimester, when levels of factor VIII may rise to double that of the normal baseline value. Treatment with coagulation factor concentrate is only rarely required during pregnancy in carriers of haemophilia A. Coagulation factor concentrate was not required in any of 117 pregnancies in carriers of haemophilia in a retrospective study from Sweden, although four mothers required a blood transfusion after delivery.[8] In another study from London, factor VIII was given during pregnancy in only one of 48 pregnancies, although DDAVP (1-desamino-

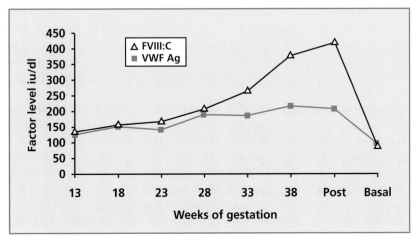

Figure 2.2 Levels of factor VIII (FVIII) and von Willebrand factor (VWF) in normal pregnancy (adapted from Stirling *et al.*[18])

8-D-arginine vasopressin; desmopressin) was given to another woman after delivery.[1] By contrast, factor IX levels do not rise significantly in pregnancy and thus carriers of haemophilia B with a low baseline factor IX level are more likely to require haemostatic support to cover delivery, particularly if caesarean section is required.

If treatment is required in carriers of either haemophilia A or B, recombinant (genetically engineered) products should be regarded as the products of choice. Plasma-derived products, including those subjected to dual-inactivation processes, have the potential to transmit parvovirus. While not normally a serious infection in non-immunocompromised adults, infection of the fetus may result in hydrops fetalis and fetal death. DDAVP is of potential value in these cases, as it can boost the plasma levels of VWF and factor VIII in the blood.[9] However, the manufacturers advise that it should be used with caution during pregnancy. Although DDAVP is theoretically a V_2 agonist devoid of action on smooth muscle, there are case reports of premature labour and hyponatraemia associated with seizures which appear to have been precipitated by intravenous infusion to pregnant women with von Willebrand's disorder (VWD).[10] However, anecdotal but unpublished experience with DDAVP in pregnancy suggests that such adverse events are rare, and DDAVP should not be regarded as absolutely contraindicated in pregnancy. DDAVP may be used after delivery, when the umbilical cord has been clamped. It does not pass into breast milk in significant amounts, and so may be given to breastfeeding mothers. DDAVP does not boost the level of factor IX in the blood and thus is of no value in carriers of haemophilia B.

Although the precise status of the fetus with regard to haemophilia may not have been established through antenatal testing, ultrasound examination to determine the fetal sex during pregnancy is strongly recommended. This may influence decisions in the management of the actual delivery: if the fetus is female it will not have a low factor VIII level. Even if the mother does not wish to know the result, it is important that this information is available to the obstetrician at the time of delivery.

In the past, caesarean section was often carried out when there was suspicion that a fetus had inherited haemophilia. This is not necessary; vaginal delivery is safe even when the fetus is known to have haemophilia, assuming there are no obstetric contraindications.[8] Epidural anaesthesia is permitted if the factor level is more than 40 iu/dl and caesarean section for obstetric reasons may be carried out without haemostatic support if the factor level is more than 50 iu/dl. Intramuscular injections should not be given.

Although it is clear that the risk of intracranial bleeding after a normal vaginal delivery is low,[11] it is a recognised complication and consideration should be given to performing an ultrasound scan of the brain to exclude this possibility. Coagulation factors VIII and IX do not cross the placenta and so a fetus would not be protected by infusion of the mother with coagulation factor concentrates during delivery. There is a case report of infusion of recombinant factor VIII by cordocentesis at the onset of labour to cover delivery.[12] It is not necessary as a routine to administer a prophylactic dose of coagulation factor concentrate to a haemophilic neonate after a normal vaginal delivery. However, it is advisable to give an infusion of a coagulation factor concentrate if instruments have been used to assist delivery; recombinant products should be regarded as the treatment of choice in such circumstances. Vacuum (Ventouse) extraction should be avoided, as the use of this instrument is associated with a high risk of cephalhaematoma or intracranial bleeding. Application of a fetal scalp electrode to monitor the fetal heart rate during labour is also best avoided, particularly since external monitoring may be used as an alternative.

After delivery, a cord blood sample should be obtained for coagulation factor assay. This opportunity should not be lost. All too frequently, a cord blood sample is not taken and this necessitates subsequent venepuncture, which may be traumatic, may result in severe bruising or bleeding and may require treatment with blood products. Only 0.5–1 ml of blood, collected in a citrated tube, is required for factor assay; there is no need to send a larger sample, which may exacerbate any anaemia in the baby. If it is routine practice to administer vitamin K by intramuscular injection, this should be withheld, or given orally, until the result of the factor assay is known.

There is a risk of postpartum haemorrhage. It is wise to check the factor level a few days after delivery. Maternal haemostatic support may be needed for 4–5 days postpartum; DDAVP may be useful.

von Willebrand's disorder

Von Willebrand factor (VWF) is a protein encoded on chromosome 12 and synthesised in endothelial cells. VWF binds to collagen and to platelets through the platelet glycoprotein Ib receptor and is essential for platelet adhesion to endothelial cells. VWF also binds circulating factor VIII noncovalently and protects it from degradation and uptake into endothelial cells. Deficiency of VWF typically results in easy bruising, prolonged bleeding from cuts and scratches, epistaxis and menorrhagia.

Much of what has been said above about pregnancy in women who are carriers of haemophilia also applies to women with VWD. It is important to establish both the type and plasma levels of factor VIII and VWF for the management of pregnant women with VWD. The level of VWF may not rise significantly during the first or even second trimester and therefore an early miscarriage may be accompanied by significant bleeding. However, the level of VWF usually rises to within the normal range by the third trimester and haemostatic support is rarely needed. Approximately 80% of all cases of von Willebrand's disorder are of the type 1 subtype, characterised by low plasma levels of VWF but qualitatively normal multimers. A concentrate of recombinant VWF is not yet available but DDAVP (desmopressin) is of potential value in these cases, as this chemical can boost the plasma levels of VWF and factor VIII in the blood.[9] The manufacturers advise that DDAVP should be used with caution during pregnancy (see above). As a general rule, normal vaginal delivery and epidural anaesthesia can be allowed with a factor VIII level (often used as a surrogate marker for VWF levels) of > 40 iu/dl, and caesarean section with a factor VIII level of >50 iu/dl.

DDAVP is of no value in the other types (2A, 2B and 3) of von Willebrand's disorder, which account for approximately 20% of cases encountered. Type 2B may be associated with mild progressive thrombocytopenia, which may lead to the first identification of the disorder. The VWF level in severe (type 3) disorder does not rise significantly in pregnancy. If haemostatic support is required in such cases, plasma-derived concentrates, which contain VWF, will be required: there is no concentrate of recombinant VWF. High-purity (including recombinant) factor VIII concentrates contain little or no VWF and are of no value. Cryoprecipitate also contains VWF, but as it not subjected to virucidal treatment (e.g. heat treatment) it is not used to treat von Willebrand's disorder in developed countries.

Several studies have documented a significantly increased risk of both primary and secondary postpartum haemorrhage in women with von Willebrand's disorder, which appears to be higher than in carriers of haemophilia.[13–15] The risk appears from these studies to be relatively higher in women with type 2 disorder than with the more common type 1. It is thus prudent to check the VWF level in all women with von Willebrand's disorder a few days after delivery: an infusion of DDAVP may be indicated where the level falls significantly soon after delivery. DDAVP does not pass in significant quantities into breast milk and is therefore safe for breastfeeding mothers.

Antenatal diagnosis of von Willebrand's disorder is not usually required or requested as the bleeding tendency is relatively mild. The disorder is inherited as an autosomal dominant condition, and thus children of either sex may inherit the condition. Severe (type 3) disorder may be readily diagnosed after birth from an umbilical cord blood sample. However, it is almost impossible to diagnose the much more common milder forms of the disorder in a neonate as the level of VWF rises significantly during birth and an apparently normal result may thus mask a mild form of disease. Testing is therefore best deferred for some months, unless surgery or some other invasive procedure is necessary. It should also be borne in mind that the expression of VWF is affected by the blood group (those with group O having the lowest levels, and those with group AB having the highest) and this can result in variable penetrance of the phenotype in a given family (in contrast with haemophilia, where the phenotype or severity of the haemophilia remains constant within a given kindred).

Other congenital bleeding disorders

Women with congenital deficiencies of other coagulation factors may be encountered occasionally.

Fibrinogen (factor I) is a 340 kD protein encoded on chromosome 4 and synthesised in hepatocytes. Fibrinogen is converted to fibrin through the action of thrombin during the process of coagulation. Fibrinogen is also essential for aggregation of platelets. Afibrinogenaemia may be associated with menorrhagia, recurrent abortion and postpartum haemorrhage. However, regular substitution treatment with infusions of fibrinogen concentrate (aiming for a trough fibrinogen level of 1 g/l) may result in a successful outcome.[16]

Factor XI is a serine protease inhibitor, encoded by a gene on chromosome 4, synthesised in hepatocytes. Deficiency of factor XI is associated with a bleeding tendency but the correlation between the plasma level and the severity of haemorrhagic manifestations is poor. Levels of less than 15% are likely to be associated with a bleeding tendency, but postoperative bleeding may be seen even in patients with only modest deficiency and levels between 50–70 iu/dl. Factor XI deficiency is particularly common among Ashkenazi Jews, but has also been reported in other many ethnic groups. Menorrhagia is a frequent problem in women with factor XI deficiency. The level of factor XI does not rise during pregnancy, in contrast to many other coagulation factors. In view of the unpredictable nature of the bleeding tendency and the poor correlation with the plasma level of factor XI, labour and delivery should be managed with caution in a centre where fresh frozen plasma can be given promptly if required. In one study of 28 pregnancies in 11 women with factor XI deficiency, the incidence of primary postpartum haemorrhage was 16%.[15] Prophylactic infusion of plasma may be required, for example to cover caesarean section. Cryoprecipitate does not contain factor XI but a lyophilised plasma-derived concentrate of factor XI is available, which has the advantage of having been subjected to a virucidal treatment such as heat treatment. However, this advantage should be balanced against the apparent thrombogenicity of the concentrate and this material is probably best reserved for severely deficient women; the post-infusion level should be monitored and maintained below 100 iu/dl.

Factor XIII enhances the stability of fibrin clots by forging covalent bonds between adjacent strands of monomeric fibrin. Congenital deficiency of this protein is rare, but is associated with a serious bleeding tendency and poor wound healing. Early reports in the literature suggested that women with factor XIII deficiency were prone to infertility and recurrent miscarriages. However, a programme of prophylaxis with monthly infusions of factor XIII concentrate is now usually initiated as soon as the condition is diagnosed in childhood and so this problem does not arise. Continued monthly infusions of factor XIII concentrate, aiming for a trough level of not less than 1.5%, is likely to result in a successful outcome in pregnancy.[17]

Key points

- Prepregnancy: genetic evaluation; immunisation against hepatitis A and B. A trial of DDAVP may be considered if baseline (nonpregnant) levels of factor VIII and/or von Willebrand factor are low.

- Good liaison is essential between haemophilia centre and obstetricians, who may be based in a different hospital.

- Baseline factor VIII (and/or IX and VWF level) should be checked at booking and in the third trimester (ideally at around 34 weeks).

- Fetal sex should be determined by ultrasound and the results should be available to the obstetrician at the time of delivery.

- Caesarean section is not routinely indicated merely because of possible haemophilia.

- Caesarean section required for obstetric reasons may be carried out without haemostatic support if the factor level is more than 50 iu/dl.

- Epidural anaesthesia is permitted if the factor level is more than 40 iu/dl. Avoid intramuscular analgesia.

- Avoid the use of fetal scalp electrodes for monitoring during labour.

- Avoid vacuum extraction (Ventouse delivery).

- Check the cord factor level after birth.

- Avoid intramuscular vitamin K until the factor result is known (although it may be given orally as an alternative).

- Give recombinant products to the baby if forceps are applied (but not routinely otherwise).

- Special observations of the baby may be warranted after delivery, including ultrasound examination of the head to exclude intracranial bleeding.

- Be aware of the risk of delayed postpartum haemorrhage. Factor levels should be monitored and haemostatic support may be required for a few days after delivery.

References

1 Kadir RA, Economides DL, Braithwaite J, Goldman E, Lee CA. The obstetric experience of carriers of haemophilia. *Br J Obstet Gynaecol* 1997;104:803–10.

2 Tedgård U, Ljung R, McNeil, TF. Reproductive choices of haemophilia carriers. *Br J Haematol* 1999;106:421–6.

3 Firth HV, Boyd PA, Chamberlain P, MacKenzie IZ, Lindenbaum RH, Huson SM. Severe limb abnormalities after chorion villus sampling at 56-66 days' gestation. *Lancet* 1991;337:762–3.

4 Firth HV, Boyd PA, Chamberlain PF, MacKenzie IZ, Morriss-Kay GM, Huson SM. Analysis of limb reduction defects in babies exposed to chorionic villus sampling. *Lancet* 1994;343:1069–71.

5 Cheung M-C, Goldberg JD, Kan YW. Prenatal diagnosis of sickle cell anaemia and thalassaemia by analysis of fetal blood cells in maternal blood. *Nat Genet* 1996;14:264–8.

6 Forestier F, Daffos F, Rainaut M, Sole Y, Amiral J. Vitamin dependent proteins in fetal hemostasis at mid trimester pregnancy. *Thromb Haemost* 1985;53:401–3.

7 Forestier F, Daffos F, Galactéros F, Bardakjian J, Rainaut M, Beuzard Y. Hematological values of 163 normal fetuses between 18 and 30 weeks of gestation. *Pediatr Res* 1986;20:342–6.

8 Ljung R, Lidgren A-C, Petrini P, Tengborn L. Normal vaginal delivery is to be recommended for haemophilia carrier gravidae. *Acta Paediatr* 1994;83:609–11.

9 Mannucci PM. Desmopressin (DDAVP) in the treatment of bleeding disorders: the first 20 years. *Blood* 1997;90:2515–21.

10 Chediak JR, Alban G, Maxey B. von Willebrand's disease and pregnancy: Management during delivery and outcome of offspring. *Am J Obstet Gynecol* 1986;155:618–24.

11 Yoffe G, Buchanan GR. Intracranial hemorrhage in newborn and young infants with hemophilia. *J Pediatr* 1988;113:333–6.

12 Gilchrist GS, Wilke JL, Muehlenbein LR, Danilenko-Dixon D. Intrauterine correction of factor VIII (FVIII) deficiency. *Haemophilia* 2001;7:497–9.

13 Ramsahoye BH, Davies SV, Dasani H, Pearson JF. Obstetric management of von Willebrand's disease: a report of 24 cases and a review of the literature. *Haemophilia* 1995;1:140–44.

14 Greer IA, Lowe GDO, Walker JJ, Forbes CD. Haemorrhagic problems in obstetrics and gynaecology in patients with congenital coagulopathies. *Br J Obstet Gynaecol* 1991;98:909–18.

15 Kadir RA, Lee CA, Sabin CA, Pollard D, Economides DL. Pregnancy in women with von Willebrand's disease or factor XI deficiency. *Br J Obstet Gynaecol* 1998;105:314–21.

16 Grech H, Majumdar G, Lawrie AS, Savidge GF. Pregnancy in congenital afibrinogenaemia: report of a successful case and review of the literature. *Br J Haematol* 1991;78:571–82.

17 Burrows RF, Ray JG, Burrows EA. Bleeding risk and reproductive capacity among patients with factor XIII deficiency: a case presentation and review of the literature. *Obstet Gynecol Surv* 2000;55:103–8.

18 Stirling Y, Woolf L, North WRS, Seghatchian MJ, Meade TW. Haemostasis in normal pregnancy. *Thromb Haemost* 1984;52:176–82.

3 Maternal and fetal thrombocytopenia

Thrombocytopenia in the mother and fetus is a common problem. This chapter reviews its causes, clinical significance, investigation and management.

The platelet count in an uncomplicated pregnancy

The maternal platelet count tends to decrease by about 10% during pregnancy with the fall being most pronounced in the last trimester.[1,2]

Maternal thrombocytopenia

The overall incidence of maternal thrombocytopenia (platelet count $<150 \times 10^9/l$) is 6–7%.[3] Incidental thrombocytopenia of pregnancy (or benign gestational thrombocytopenia) is the most frequent cause of maternal thrombocytopenia (74%), followed by hypertensive disorders of pregnancy (21%) and immune causes (4%). Less common causes include thrombotic microangiopathies, such as thrombotic thrombocytopenic purpura and haemolytic uraemic syndrome, and bone marrow failure due to a primary haematological disorder.

Incidental thrombocytopenia of pregnancy

There is typically mild thrombocytopenia with a platelet count in the range $70–150 \times 10^9/l$. It starts in the second trimester, is most marked at the time of delivery, and is diagnosed by excluding other causes. It is probably a more pronounced form of the 'physiological' fall in the platelet count in uncomplicated pregnancies described above. The pathogenesis is not well understood, but is probably due to the combined effects of haemodilution and increased nonimmune platelet destruction.

There is no clinical impact on the mother or fetus. The maternal platelet count returns to normal within 6 weeks of delivery. Management merely involves observing the platelet count, and avoiding any unnecessary intervention.

Hypertensive disorders of pregnancy

Hypertensive disease in pregnancy remains one of the leading causes of direct maternal mortality.[4] Thrombocytopenia complicating hypertensive disorders of pregnancy is responsible for about 20% of cases of maternal thrombocytopenia. Up to 50% of women with pre-eclampsia develop thrombocytopenia. It is usually mild or moderate, although occasionally it may be severe, and is usually proportional to the severity of the pre-eclampsia. The nadir of the platelet count is often after delivery; the platelet count returns to normal within a week after delivery. The cause of thrombocytopenia in pre-eclampsia is unknown but is thought to be due to increased platelet consumption, perhaps associated with binding of platelets to damaged endothelium.

The HELLP syndrome is part of the spectrum of hypertensive disorders of pregnancy, and is characterised by haemolysis, elevated liver function tests and low platelets. The degree of thrombocytopenia correlates with the degree of abnormalities in liver enzymes and can be used as a marker of the severity of HELLP. As in pre-eclampsia, the nadir of the platelet count is often 1–2 days after delivery with a further 2–3 days before it returns to normal.

Fifty-seven percent of hypertension-related maternal deaths in the latest Confidential Enquiries into Maternal Deaths (CEMD)[5] report were associated with HELLP syndrome either before delivery or with further rapid clinical deterioration after delivery. Many women with HELLP syndrome do not meet the criteria for severe pre-eclampsia in terms of blood pressure recordings or significant proteinuria. More commonly they present with malaise, epigastric pain, nausea with or without vomiting, and right upper quadrant tenderness. Hypertension and proteinuria often occur after the presentation of HELLP.

Management will be largely gestation-dependent, with most advocating urgent delivery if the pregnancy is viable. At early gestation, some advocate the use of steroids to prolong the pregnancy. Platelet transfusions should be avoided unless there is severe thrombocytopenic bleeding because they may increase the risk of thrombotic events, which can occur in this condition.[6,7]

Disseminated intravascular coagulation

The pregnancy-related causes of disseminated intravascular coagulation (DIC) include pre-eclampsia, placental abruption, amniotic fluid embolism and, rarely, retention of a dead fetus. Management is similar to the management of DIC from other causes and usually involves delivery and the use of blood components (fresh frozen plasma and platelet transfusions) in the presence of bleeding and abnormal coagulation. Early involvement of a consultant haematologist and a consultant obstetrician is essential as soon as a coagulation problem has been identified. Obstetric interventions will depend on the clinical situation but early delivery, once the coagulation problem has been corrected sufficiently to allow operative delivery, is generally required.

Immune thrombocytopenia

Immune thrombocytopenia is responsible for about 4% of maternal thrombocytopenia. Most cases are due to idiopathic autoimmune thrombocytopenia, but some are drug-related and some associated with HIV infection. Diagnosis is largely one of exclusion of other causes of thrombocytopenia; platelet antibody testing is not sufficiently sensitive or specific to make a definitive diagnosis of immune thrombocytopenia in individual cases, and is of no proven value in predicting the fetal or neonatal platelet count. The following recommendations for management come from guidelines drawn up by the British Committee for Standards in Haematology (BCSH) on behalf of the British Society for Haematology.[8,9]

If the maternal platelet count is >50 x 10^9/l:

- monitor the platelet count every 2 weeks
- vaginal delivery allowed
- avoid epidural anaesthesia if the platelet count is <80 x 10^9/l.

If the maternal platelet count is <50 x 10^9/l:

- increased risk of bleeding at delivery
- raise the platelet count to >50 x 10^9/l for vaginal delivery
- raise the platelet count to >80 x 10^9/l for caesarean section
- treatment may be required earlier in pregnancy if the mother has bleeding, which is usually associated with a platelet count <20 x 10^9/l.

Treatment options are steroids or high-dose intravenous immuno-globulin G (IVIgG), but no comparative trials of steroids and IVIgG have been published. The precise mode of action of corticosteroids is due to a combination of inhibition of reticuloendothelial destruction of antibody-coated platelets and reduced antibody synthesis. The mechanism of action of IVIgG primarily involves blockade of Fc receptors on macrophages so that antibody-coated platelets are not removed from the circulation by the reticuloendothelial system.

If the duration of treatment is likely to be short, that is, in the third trimester, the use of prednisolone (initial dose 1 mg/kg/day based on prepregnancy weight) is a cost-effective approach. The dose of steroids should be reduced to a level that maintains the platelet count at a level which prevents bleeding. Patients should be monitored for adverse effects such as hypertension, hyperglycaemia, osteoporosis, excessive weight gain and psychosis. Ninety percent of the dose of a steroid is metabolised by the placenta so fetal adverse effects such as adrenal suppression are unlikely.

If treatment is likely to be prolonged, or there is a need for an unacceptably high dose of steroids, IVIgG should be considered (0.4 g/kg/day for 5 days is the standard dose, although 1 g/kg/day for 2 days is probably as effective and is more convenient). The response rate (about 80%) and duration of response (about 2–3 weeks) are similar to that in nonpregnant women. After an initial course, single infusions can be used to prevent bleeding and ensure that there is a satisfactory platelet count before delivery. Other immunosuppressive drugs which are frequently used for immune thrombocytopenia in nonpregnant women should be avoided in pregnancy.

It is not possible accurately to predict the fetal platelet count from the mother's platelet count or history. Invasive fetal procedures such as cordocentesis and scalp blood sampling are not recommended and the use of fetal scalp electrodes and the Ventouse should be avoided. Caesarean section is only recommended for obstetric indications. The baby's platelet count should be measured on a cord sample after delivery, and if thrombocytopenia is detected the count should be monitored closely for the next 5 days as it is likely to fall further. If the platelet count is $<20 \times 10^9$/l or if there is bleeding, treatment with high-dose IVIgG (1 g/kg) usually produces a rapid response.

Fetal and neonatal thrombocytopenia

The normal platelet count in the fetus and in the neonate is the same as in adults. Neonatal thrombocytopenia has many causes (Table 3.1), and is the most common haematological problem in the newborn infant, and probably the fetus as well. A platelet count of $<150 \times 10^9$/l occurs in about 1% of unselected neonates, and of $<50 \times 10^9$/l in 0.12%.[3]

Between 40% and 72% of low-birthweight neonates admitted to neonatal intensive care units have thrombocytopenia.[10,11] The mechanism of the thrombocytopenia is often multifactorial, frequently involving sepsis and hypoxia. Management is primarily that of the underlying medical problems, but also includes platelet transfusions to prevent severe thrombocytopenia (platelet count $<50 \times 10^9$/l) and bleeding.[12]

Neonatal alloimmune thrombocytopenia

Neonatal alloimmune thrombocytopenia (NAIT) is the most important cause of severe fetal and neonatal thrombocytopenia, both because of its frequency and the bleeding associated with it.[3] A cord platelet count of $<20 \times 10^9$/l is usually due to NAIT.

NAIT is the platelet equivalent of haemolytic disease of the newborn, and is due to fetomaternal incompatibility for human platelet antigens (HPA). About 80% of serologically proven cases are due to anti-HPA-1a (or PlA1 in the old nomenclature for platelet antigens), 15% due to anti-HPA-5b and 5% due to other platelet antibody specificities.[13] There is no routine antenatal screening for NAIT. Most cases are diagnosed after birth, but the condition develops *in utero* and the fetus may be severely affected. Unlike haemolytic disease of the newborn, nearly 50% of cases occur in the first pregnancy.

The incidence of NAIT is between one in 1000 and one in 1500 pregnancies. It is surprising that its incidence is so low given that 2% of women are HPA-1a negative and that the majority of them will be carrying a HPA-1a positive fetus. However, only a minority of HPA-1a negative pregnant women (around 10%) will develop anti-HPA-1a, and

---

Table 3.1 Causes of neonatal thrombocytopenia

Increased platelet destruction

Immune-mediated:
  Neonatal alloimmune thrombocytopenia
  Neonatal thrombocytopenia due to maternal autoantibodies
Platelet consumption:
  Maternal eclampsia/HELLP syndrome
  Disseminated intravascular coagulation
  Giant haemangiomas (Kasabach–Merritt syndrome)

Decreased platelet production

Amegakaryocytic thrombocytopenia, e.g. thrombocytopenia-absent-radius (TAR) syndrome
Wiskott–Aldrich syndrome
Marrow infiltration e.g. leukaemia, neuroblastoma
Osteopetrosis

Mixed origin

Infection:
  Congenital, e.g. TORCH syndrome
  Acquired, e.g. bacterial sepsis

Miscellaneous

Exchange transfusion
Haemolytic disease of the newborn
Chromosome abnormalities, e.g. Down syndrome

---

only a proportion of those will have a clinically affected baby.[14] The reason for the low level of HPA-1a alloimmunisation is the close association with a certain human leucocyte antigen (HLA) type (HLA DRB3*0101, which is present in about 30% of individuals). Only a proportion (about 30%) of HPA-1a women with this HLA type develop anti-HPA-1a.

NAIT is usually suspected in babies with bleeding or unexplained isolated thrombocytopenia. The clinical diagnosis is one of exclusion: the infant has no signs of DIC, infection or congenital anomalies known to be associated with thrombocytopenia, and the mother has had a normal pregnancy with no history of autoimmune disease, thrombocytopenia or drugs which may cause thrombocytopenia. While 65% of cases of NAIT have an uneventful outcome, it has been reported that 25% either die or have long-term neurological disability because of intracranial haemorrhage. Although severe haemorrhage is most likely to occur during or soon after delivery, about 50% of intracranial haemorrhages occur spontaneously *in utero* (Figure 3.1).

Unfortunately, some cases of NAIT are not detected until there has been a careful review of the obstetric history as demonstrated by Case History 1, where it was not until a thorough examination of the post-mortem reports had been undertaken at the time of pre-conception counselling that the possibility of NAIT was raised, and the mother found to be HPA-1a negative and to have anti-HPA-1a. In Case History 2, the

---

CASE HISTORY 1
- 30-year-old para 2 + 4:
    1. early termination of pregnancy
    2. term pregnancy, normal delivery, female alive and well
    3. early termination of pregnancy
    4. termination of pregnancy 21 weeks – Dandy Walker malformation
    5. early embryonic loss
    6. intrauterine death 32 weeks
- Initially referred for preconception counselling. Review of postmortem reports from pregnancies 4 and 6 showed that both were due to intracranial haemorrhage. Platelet antibodies were tested and HPA-1a antibodies found.
- In a subsequent pregnancy IVIgG was administered from 15 weeks of gestation and the first FBS performed at 21 of weeks gestation. The initial fetal platelet count was 11×10^9/l, indicating severe disease.
- After a series of weekly transfusions the baby was delivered by emergency caesarean section and is alive and well.

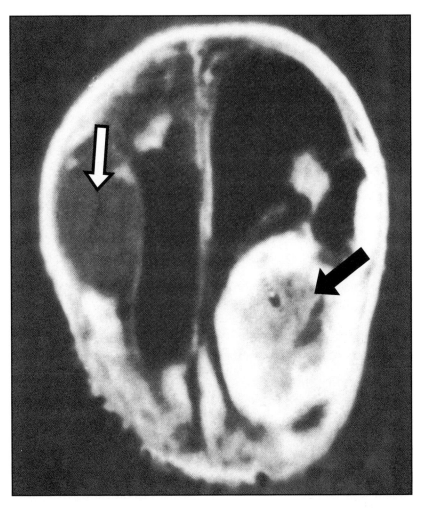

Figure 3.1 MRI studies on a neonate delivered at 32 weeks of gestation following the observation of intracranial haemorrhage in a pregnancy known to be affected by alloimmune throbocytopenia due to anti-HPA-1a showing subacute haematoma (arrow) and chronic haematoma (open arrow) (from De Vries *et al.*[31])

diagnosis of NAIT was not suspected until the observation of hydrocephalus in the fifth pregnancy affected by late miscarriage at 17–18 weeks of gestation.

Optimal management of NAIT depends on rapid diagnosis and prompt transfusion of compatible platelet concentrates to babies who are severely thrombocytopenic or who are bleeding.[8] There is no need to wait for platelet antibody identification in suspected cases. HPA-1a and 5b negative platelet concentrates should be used initially because more than 90% of severe cases of NAIT are due to anti-HPA-1a or anti-HPA-5b.[15] The National Blood Service maintains a stock at all times. The thrombocytopenia usually resolves within 2 weeks although it may last as long as 6 weeks. A cerebral ultrasound should be carried out to determine if intracranial haemorrhage has occurred.

The management of subsequent pregnancies in women with a previous affected pregnancy is problematic. In general, thrombocytopenia of equal or greater severity will occur in over 85% of subsequent pregnancies. The aim of management is to prevent severe bleeding both *in utero* and during and after delivery. Before a subsequent pregnancy, the father's platelets should be typed to determine if all infants will have the target antigen. If the father is HPA-1a/1a, all subsequent pregnancies by that partner will be affected. If the father is HPA-1a/1b, the fetal platelet type should be determined as there is a 50% chance that the baby is HPA-1b/1b and unaffected.

The presence or absence of haemorrhage and its severity in a previous pregnancy are the best guides to the risk of bleeding in subsequent pregnancies.[16] Noninvasive measures such as levels of maternal platelet antibodies are not predictive of the severity of thrombocytopenia or the risk of haemorrhage.

There is a continuing debate about the optimal antenatal management of NAIT and how best to define the response to treatment. Early caesarean section alone is not considered to be effective in preventing antenatal or perinatal haemorrhage. The therapeutic options are the maternal administration of high-dose IVIgG (1 g/kg/week) with or without steroids,[17] or the use of serial (weekly) fetal platelet transfusions without maternal treatment.[18] For both approaches to antenatal management, fetal blood sampling (FBS) has been used for initial assessment of the fetal platelet count, for administration of platelet transfusions and for the monitoring of the effectiveness of treatment.

The response rate to maternal therapy with high-dose IVIgG, with or without steroids, is about 70%.[17] The use of serial platelet transfusions more reliably increases the fetal platelet count (see Case histories 2 and 3) but at the risk of a higher complication rate associated with repeated FBS.[19,20] Other studies support the approach of initial therapy with maternally administered IVIgG without FBS to assess the pretreatment fetal platelet count.[21,22] The commencement of maternal therapy can be stratified on the basis of the severity of the sibling history of NAIT, beginning at 12–16 weeks of gestation when there has been antenatal intracranial haemorrhage in a previous pregnancy and at 20 weeks of gestation in the absence of severe haemorrhage in previous pregnancies. There is no consensus about the value of FBS to assess the response to IVIgG, although it is our practice to do this 8 weeks after the initiation of IVIgG to detect non-responders. These cases can be treated by doubling the dose of IVIgG to 2g/kg/week, adding prednisolone (0.5 mg/kg/day) or switching to weekly fetal platelet transfusions. FBS at 2–4 week intervals is needed to assess the response to more aggressive medical treatment. Antenatal treatment appears to have the potential to improve the outcome of severely affected cases of NAIT but there is little information on the long-term development of children who have been treated *in utero*.

There is increasing interest in antenatal screening for NAIT because of improvements in antenatal management and a greater awareness of the frequency of antenatal haemorrhage and its consequences.[23] Studies have demonstrated the feasibility of large-scale antenatal testing of mothers for their HPA-1a type and the presence of HPA-1a antibodies using the antenatal samples sent for red cell serology.[24] There remain some problems to be resolved before considering the introduction of routine antenatal screening for NAIT, such as:

- the uncertainty about the optimal management of women with anti-HPA-1a with no previous history of affected pregnancies, and the recognition that FBS has significant risks
- the lack of reliable methods for predicting the severity of NAIT and identifying those pregnancies at greatest risk of antenatal haemorrhage where antenatal intervention might be justified.

SPECIFICATION FOR PLATELETS FOR INTRAUTERINE TRANSFUSION

Donor:

- HPA type compatible with maternal antibodies, usually HPA-1a negative
- Group O RhD negative for the first transfusion (for subsequent transfusions, ABO and RhD group of the donor should be compatible with the fetal blood group)
- no HPA or HLA antibodies
- no high titre ABO antibodies.

Platelet concentrates:

- high concentration of platelets (usually in the range 2.5–3.0 x 10^{12}/l compared with 1.4 x 10^{12}/l for standard platelet concentrates for use in neonates or adults) to reduce the volume of the transfusion. The hyperconcentrates are prepared using a modification of the procedure for collection of platelet concentrates by apheresis[30]
- gamma-irradiated to prevent transfusion-associated graft-versus-host disease
- cytomegalovirus-seronegative
- leucocyte-depleted
- transfuse within 24 hours of collection.

Technical aspects of fetal blood sampling

The technique employed for transabdominal ultrasound guided FBS and intravascular transfusion and the risks involved have been well documented elsewhere[25-27] and are the same as for red cell allo-immunisation. Whereas in haemolytic disease of the newborn the needle may be removed while the haematocrit is estimated before transfusion is commenced, in NAIT this is not feasible, because removal of the needle from the umbilical cord in the presence of a low platelet count can result in rapid exsanguination of the fetus. For this reason, in every instance that FBS is performed in NAIT a prophylactic platelet transfusion is performed in order to protect the fetus from exsanguination, and intraperitoneal transfusion of platelets is never performed.

From 26 weeks of gestation, FBS and platelet transfusion should be performed in the operating theatre, where facilities are available to perform an emergency caesarean section should there be signs of fetal distress or bleeding from the sampling site. Unpublished data from the Oxford Rhesus Therapy Unit indicate that there is approximately a 4% chance of rapid delivery being required at the time of each transfusion.

The volume of platelet hyperconcentrate to be transfused is calculated from the formula: Volume of concentrate = (desired platelet increment x fetoplacental blood volume for gestational age) x R ÷ platelet count of the concentrate, which is measured on each occasion.[18]

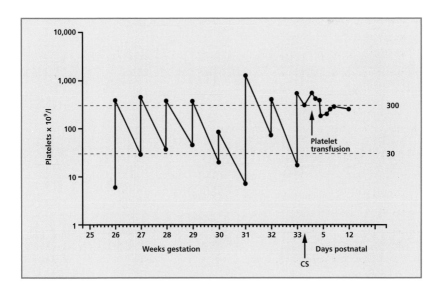

Figure 3.2 Fetal platelet transfusion

The fetoplacental blood volume for gestational age is calculated from standard charts. The immediate post-transfusion platelet increment was found to be 50% of that expected, that is 50% platelet recovery, probably because of pooling in the fetoplacental circulation.[28] The volume calculation takes account of this by introducing the factor R = 2, thus doubling the volume of platelets transfused.

The strategy for serial fetal platelet transfusions in NAIT is shown in Figure 3.2. If the fetal platelet count is raised to 300–500 x 10^9/l after each transfusion, it is usually no lower than 30 x 10^9/l one week later.[29] This may be considered a 'safe' level at which to maintain the fetal platelet count, and 7 days an acceptable interval between transfusions in the high risk pregnancies where serial transfusions are used. If the interval between transfusions is prolonged beyond 7 days, the nadir of the fetal platelet count is less than 30 x 10^9/l.

Summary

The optimal care of thrombocytopenia in pregnancy requires a close working relationship between obstetrician, paediatrician and haematologist. A better understanding of the risks of thrombocytopenia in pregnancy to the mother and fetus has resulted in better targeting of treatment: withholding it in low-risk situations and using intensive therapy where there is high risk.

Key points

- The most common causes of maternal thrombocytopenia are benign gestational thrombocytopenia (74%), which has no clinical significance for mother or fetus, pre-eclampsia (21%) and immune causes (4%).

- If necessary in maternal immune thrombocytopenia, the platelet count can be raised with steroid or immunoglobulin (IVIgG) therapy, or platelets given for acute situations.

- There is an increased risk of bleeding with low platelet counts. Epidural anaesthesia and caesarean section should be avoided if the platelet count is $<80 \times 10^9/l$; vaginal delivery is allowed if the platelet count is $>50 \times 10^9/l$.

- Invasive fetal procedures such as cordocentesis and scalp blood sampling, and use of fetal scalp electrodes and the Ventouse should be avoided. The baby's platelet count should be measured on a cord sample after delivery.

- Neonatal alloimmune thrombocytopenia may be associated with fetal or neonatal intracranial haemorrhage; severe neonatal thrombocytopenia should be treated with transfusion of compatible platelet concentrate and cerebral ultrasound should be performed.

- Management of subsequent pregnancy after NAIT has been diagnosed should include paternal platelet typing to determine the chance (50% or 100%) of carrying an affected fetus.

- Maternal treatment with high-dose IVIgG, beginning at 12–20 weeks of gestation, is the current preferred approach to antenatal management.

References

1   Boehlen F, Hohlfeld P, Extermann P, Perneger TV, de Moerloose P. Platelet count at term pregnancy: a reappraisal of the threshold. *Obstet Gynecol* 2000;95:29–33.

2   Sainio S, Kekomaki R, Riikonen S, Teramo K. Maternal thrombocytopenia at term: a population-based study. *Acta Obstet Gynecol Scand* 2000;79:744–9.

3   Burrows RF, Kelton JG. Fetal thrombocytopenia and its relation to maternal thrombocytopenia. *N Engl J Med* 1993;329:1463–6.

4   Lewis G. Introduction and key findings 2000–2002. In: Lewis G, editor. *Why Mothers Die 2000–2002. The Sixth Report of the Confidential Enquiries into Maternal Deaths in the United Kingdom.* London: RCOG Press; 2004. p. 25–58.

5   Neilson JP. Pre-eclampsia and eclampsia. In: Lewis G, editor. *Why Mothers Die 2000–2002. The Sixth Report of the Confidential Enquiries into Maternal Deaths in the United Kingdom.* London: RCOG Press; 2004. p. 79–85.

6   Magann EF, Bass D, Chauhan SP, Sullivan Dl, Martin RW, Martin JN Jr. Antepartum corticosteroids: disease stabilization in patients with the syndrome of hemolysis, elevated liver enzymes, and low platelets (HELLP). *Am J Obstet Gynecol* 1994;171:1148–53.

7   Hagan A, Ebert A, Lange J, Zemlin M, Hopp H. The impact of pregnancy-prolonging management on maternal and neonatal morbidity in HELLP syndrome. *Zentalbl Gynakol* 2001;123:513–19.

8   Letsky EA, Greaves M. Guidelines on the investigation and management of thrombocytopenia in pregnancy and neonatal alloimmune thrombocytopenia. *Br J Haematol* 1996;95:21–6.

9   Provan D, Newland A, Norfolk D, *et al.* British Committee for Standards in Haematology, Working Party of the General Haematology Task Force. Guidelines for the investigation and management of idiopathic thrombocytopenic purpura in adults, children and in pregnancy. *B J Haematol* 2003;120:574–96.

10 Mehta P, Vasa R, Neumann L, Karpatkin M. Thrombocytopenia in the high-risk infant. *J Pediatr* 1980;97:791–4.

11 Murray NA, Roberts IAG. Circulating megakaryocytes and their progenitors in early thrombocytopenia in preterm neonates. *Pediatr Res* 1996;40:112–19.

12 Roberts IAG, Murray NA. Management of thrombocytopenia in neonates. *Br J Haematol* 1999;105:864–70.

13 Mueller-Eckhardt C, Kiefel V, Grubert A, et al. 348 cases of suspected neonatal alloimmune neonatal thrombocytopenia. Lancet 1989;1:363–6.

14 Williamson LM, Hackett G, Rennie J, *et al.* The natural history of fetomaternal alloimmunisation to the platelet-specific antigen HPA-1a as determined by antenatal screening. *Blood* 1998;92:2280–87.

15 Murphy MF, Verjee S, Greaves M. Inadequacies in the postnatal management of fetomaternal alloimmune thrombocytopenia. *Br J Haematol* 1999;105:123–6.

16 Bussel JB, Zabusky MR, Berkowitz Rl, McFarland JG. Fetal alloimmune thrombocytopenia. *N Engl J Med* 1997;337:22–6.

17 Bussel JB, Berkowitz RL, Lynch L, *et al.* Antenatal management of alloimmune thrombocytopenia with intravenous gamma-globulin: a randomized trial of the addition of low-dose steroid to intravenous gamma-globulin. *Am J Obstet Gynecol* 1996;174:1414–23.

18 Murphy MF, Waters AH, Doughty HA, *et al.* Antenatal management of fetomaternal alloimmune thrombocytopenia – report of 15 affected pregnancies. *Transfus Med* 1994;4:281–92.

19 Paidas MJ, Berkowitz RL, Lynch L, *et al.* Alloimmune thrombocytopenia: fetal and neonatal losses related to cordocentesis. *Am J Obstet Gynecol* 1995;172:475–9.

20 Overton TG, Duncan KR, Jolly M, Letsky E, Fisk NM. Serial aggressive platelet transfusion for fetal alloimmune thrombocytopenia: platelet dynamics and perinatal outcome. *Am J Obstet Gynecol* 2002;186:826–31.

21 Radder CM, Brand A, Kanhai HH. A less invasive treatment strategy to prevent intracranial haemorrhage in fetal and neonatal alloimmune thrombocytopenia. *Am J Obstet Gynecol* 2001;185:683–8.

22 Birchall JE, Murphy MF, Kaplan C, Kroll H, on behalf of the European FMAIT Study Group. European collaborative study of the antenatal management of feto-maternal alloimmune thrombocytopenia. *Br J Haematol* 2003;122:275–88.

23 Murphy MF, Williamson LM. Antenatal screening for fetomaternal alloimmune thrombocytopenia: an evaluation using the criteria of the National Screening Committee. *Br J Haematol* 2000;111:726–32.

24 Murphy MF, Williamson LM, Urbaniak SJ. Antenatal screening for fetomaternal alloimmune thrombocytopenia: should we be doing it? *Vox Sanguinis* 2002;83(suppl 1):409–16.

25 Bang J, Bock JE, Trolle D. Ultrasound-guided fetal intravenous transfusion for severe rhesus haemolytic disease. *BMJ (Clin Res Ed)* 1982;284:373–4.

26 Daffos F, Capella-Pavlovsky M, Forestier F. Fetal blood sampling during pregnancy with use of a needle guided by ultrasound: a study of 606 consecutive cases. *Am J Obstet Gynecol* 1985;153:655–60.

27 Weiner CP, Williamson RA, Wenstrom KD, *et al.* Management of fetal haemolytic disease by cordocentesis II. Outcome of treatment. *Am J Obstet Gynecol* 1991;165:1302–7.

28 Murphy MF, Pullon HWH, Metcalfe P, Chapman JF, Jenkins E, Waters AH, *et al.* Management of fetal alloimmune thrombocytopenia by weekly *in utero* platelet transfusions. *Vox Sanguinis* 1990;58:45–9.

29 Murphy MF, Pullon HWH, Metcalfe P, *et al.* Management of fetal alloimmune thrombocytopenia by weekly in utero platelet transfusions. *Vox Sanguinis* 1990;58:45–9.

30 Dumont LJ, Kriladsiri P, Seghatchian J, Taylor LA, Howell CA, Murphy MF. Preparation and storage characteristics of white cell-reduced high concentration platelet concentrates collected by an apheresis system for transfusion *in utero*. *Transfusion* 2000;40:91–100.

31 De Vries LS, Connell J, Bydder GM, *et al.* Recurrent intracranial haemorrhages *in utero* in an infant with alloimmune thrombocytopenia. *Br J Obstet Gynaecol* 1988;95:299–302.

4 Massive obstetric haemorrhage

Haemorrhage is a major cause of maternal mortality. In developing countries it causes about 28% (>125 000) of known maternal deaths each year; the risk is approximately one in 1000 deliveries.[1] In developed countries, antenatal ultrasonic diagnosis of placenta praevia, routine use of oxytocics in the third stage of labour, blood transfusion and intensive care have greatly reduced maternal deaths due to haemorrhage. In the UK, the maternal mortality rate is less than one in 100 000. Haemorrhage is a leading cause of these deaths. Twenty-two maternal deaths, 17 directly due to haemorrhage, and five in which haemorrhage played a significant part, were reported to the CEMD in the triennium 2000–2002.[2] Severe, possibly life-threatening, haemorrhage occurs in approximately 6.7 per 1000 deliveries in the UK.[3] Haemorrhage may also cause significant morbidity in survivors by predisposing to anaemia and infection.

Definition

Massive obstetric haemorrhage implies the loss of large, potentially life-threatening, amounts of blood from the genital tract. Various definitions have been suggested: blood loss in excess of 1000 or 1500 ml from the genital tract,[4,5] blood loss of more than 150 ml per minute, blood loss requiring immediate transfusion or transfusion of more than ten units of blood within 24 hours, or replacement of the patient's total blood volume or 50% of the circulating blood volume in less than three hours.[6] In practice, accurate measurement of blood loss is difficult and the amount and rate of bleeding is often underestimated. In some situations, such as ectopic pregnancy, placental abruption and uterine rupture, major blood loss may be partially or completely concealed with little or no external bleeding.

Causes of massive haemorrhage

Massive obstetric haemorrhage is usually due to placenta praevia, premature placental separation (abruption) or postpartum causes (Table 4.1) and is often associated with coagulopathy. Haemorrhage is often a major

Table 4.1 Deaths from haemorrhage by cause and mortality rate per million maternities; United Kingdom 1985–2002[2]

Triennium	Placental abruption	Placenta praevia	Postpartum haemorrhage	Total	Rate per million maternities
1985–87	4	0	6	10	4.4
1988–90	6	5	11	22	9.3
1991–93	3	4	8	15	6.5
1994–96	4	3	5	12	5.5
1997–99	3	3	1	7	3.3
2000–02	3	4	10	17	8.5

factor in early pregnancy deaths due to spontaneous miscarriage, termination of pregnancy and ectopic pregnancy.

Ectopic pregnancy

Most maternal deaths associated with ectopic pregnancy, which is the most common cause of death in early pregnancy, are due to haemorrhage. In 2000–2002, 11 maternal deaths due to ectopic pregnancy were reported to the CEMD.[7] The incidence of ectopic pregnancy is 1–2% of all pregnancies and is rising, probably due to the sexually transmitted spread of *Chlamydia trachomatis*, the main cause of pelvic inflammatory disease in the UK.[8] Other risk factors associated with ectopic pregnancy are shown in Table 4.2.

The rate of deaths from ectopic pregnancy is not falling. This may be partly explained by the increased incidence of the condition; however, Neilson[7] identifies the most important problem as failure to suspect ectopic

Table 4.2 Risk factors associated with ectopic pregnancy[25]

Previous pelvic inflammatory disease	x 4
Previous tubal surgery	x 4.5
Previous ectopic pregnancy	x 10
Previous sterilisation	x 9
Current progesterone IUCD use (except MIRENA)	x 10
Assisted reproduction	
Exposure to DES *in utero*	

DES = diethylstilboestrol; IUCD = intrauterine contraceptive device;
MIRENA = levonorgestrel-releasing IUCD

pregnancy and, therefore, to perform any appropriate investigations. Most ectopic pregnancies present between five and nine weeks of gestation when the woman may be unaware that she is pregnant. Many women who have died from ectopic pregnancy presented with symptoms of urinary or gastrointestinal conditions. The possibility of atypical presentation should be appreciated by all professionals likely to encounter women with ectopic pregnancy, including medical and nursing students and trainees in relevant specialties, particularly primary care, obstetrics and gynaecology, general surgery and emergency medicine.[7]

Ruptured tubal ectopic pregnancy classically presents with acute severe lower abdominal pain followed by circulatory collapse. The onset may be so sudden and intraperitoneal bleeding so severe that the woman may develop irreversible hypovolaemic shock before effective resuscitation can be commenced. Torrential bleeding can occur particularly when the ectopic site is in the uterine cornus or, rarely, the cervix. It may be impossible to resuscitate the patient without first arresting the bleeding, and immediate laparotomy (while resuscitation is proceeding) may be lifesaving. Senior medical staff, including anaesthetists, should be involved early, and difficult surgical cases should not be delegated to unsupervised junior doctors. Laparoscopic surgery for ectopic pregnancy, although associated with less blood loss, lower analgesic requirements, shorter hospital stay and quicker postoperative recovery than open surgery, should be undertaken only by appropriately trained surgeons and is not recommended when profound shock is present.[9]

Fortunately, most cases of ectopic pregnancy do not present in such a dramatic way. A history of amenorrhoea, abdominal pain and tenderness, and a small amount of vaginal bleeding is more usual. However, many women who have an ectopic pregnancy do not have pain or amenorrhoea and a high index of suspicion for ectopic pregnancy should always be maintained. Urinary dipstick tests for beta human chorionic gonado-trophin (βhCG) are sensitive to values as low as 25 miu/ml, are inexpensive, simple to use, and provide reliable results within minutes. It is recommended that dipstick testing for βhCG should be available in general practices, accident and emergency departments and specialist units in hospitals and be performed in any woman of reproductive age with unexplained abdominal pain.[7]

Antepartum haemorrhage

The main causes of antepartum haemorrhage are placenta praevia and placental abruption. Other causes include vasa praevia, marginal bleeding, heavy 'show', local lesions of the cervix, vagina and vulva, and extragenital sources.

Placenta praevia

In placenta praevia, the placenta is wholly or partially implanted in the lower uterine segment. If it encroaches on the cervical os it is termed major placenta praevia; if not, minor placenta praevia. The cause is unknown, but it is associated with increasing maternal age and parity, smoking, previous caesarean section, previous placenta praevia and previous spontaneous or induced miscarriage.[10]

Second-trimester ultrasound scan, routine in most maternity units in the UK, diagnoses many cases of asymptomatic placenta praevia. Such women, given appropriate advice, may be managed as outpatients.[10] The placental site should be reassessed later in pregnancy because, as the lower uterine segment forms, apparent upward migration of the placenta may occur. A high incidence of false positive diagnosis of placenta praevia is associated with second-trimester transabdominal ultrasound scans. A reasonably full bladder at the time of ultrasound scan is important to clearly define the anterior border of the lower uterine segment. The lower edge of a posterior placenta may be difficult to assess because of the intervening tissues, including fetal parts. Gentle transvaginal ultrasound scan is safe and is more accurate than transabdominal ultrasound in locating the placenta.[11] Colour Doppler ultrasound may also be helpful. An os–placenta distance of 3 cm or more after 20 weeks of gestation excludes placenta praevia.[12]

Classically, placenta praevia presents with painless vaginal bleeding, usually in the third trimester, due to separation of the placental edge as the lower uterine segment forms and the cervix begins to thin, shorten and dilate. The uterus is usually soft and not tender, and fetal parts are easily felt, with no disturbance of the fetal heart rate. The presenting part may be high or the fetal lie unstable. Initial bleeds are usually minor but tend to recur ('warning bleeds'); more serious haemorrhage is likely or inevitable when the cervix begins to dilate. The diagnosis of placenta praevia is confirmed by ultrasound scan. **Digital vaginal examination may precipitate major haemorrhage and should never be performed until placenta praevia has been firmly excluded.** Accurate ultrasound diagnosis of the presence and extent of placenta praevia has reduced the need for vaginal examination in theatre to assess the feasibility of vaginal delivery.

Major asymptomatic placenta praevia in the third trimester is generally managed expectantly on an inpatient basis. There is no evidence to guide the best time for admission; it may be as soon as bleeding occurs, or at some time between 34 and 37 weeks of gestation. The aim is to postpone delivery until 37 to 38 weeks of gestation; the timing of delivery has to balance fetal prematurity against the increasing risk of spontaneous labour with possible heavy bleeding as pregnancy nears term. Women known to have placenta praevia should be booked for delivery in a hospital with ready access to adequate blood transfusion services. Documented discussion between the woman, her partner and a senior obstetrician about the mode of delivery and possible complications, such as blood transfusion or caesarean hysterectomy, should take place during the antenatal period.

Placenta praevia presenting with severe haemorrhage is managed by appropriate resuscitation and caesarean section. Less severe haemorrhage may be managed expectantly and a course of steroid given to enhance fetal lung maturity. Tocolytics to reduce uterine activity may be useful.[11]

Most cases of placenta praevia are delivered by caesarean section. This can be hazardous. The lower segment is often abnormally vascular with large surface veins, especially when the placenta is anterior. It may be necessary to cut directly through the placenta, or to burrow under and separate it, before delivering the baby. Heavy bleeding may occur and may delay delivery by obscuring the operative field. Speed is important to minimise the effect of placental separation on the baby, and also to limit blood loss. A transverse fetal lie may cause difficulty in delivery. The lower uterine segment contains less muscle than the upper segment so the contraction and retraction of the uterine muscle forming the 'living ligature' of the blood vessels in the placental bed may be less efficient and allow continued bleeding. The risk of placenta accreta, increta or percreta (morbidly adherent placenta) is significant (24–67%) in women with an anterior placenta praevia and one or more previous caesarean sections.[13] If suspected, it may be possible to diagnose placenta accreta antenatally by ultrasound imaging, colour Doppler, power amplitude ultrasonic angiography or magnetic resonance imaging (MRI).[11] Blood loss can be massive in cases of morbidly adherent placenta and hysterectomy is often necessary. For all the above reasons, caesarean section for placenta praevia should always be carried out by an experienced operator and a consultant should be readily available.[2] This is particularly important in higher risk situations – emergencies, anterior placenta, previous uterine scars and placenta accreta.

Placental abruption

Placental abruption is bleeding following premature separation of a normally sited placenta, that is, one implanted entirely in the upper uterine segment. The incidence is between 0.49 and 1.8%.[14] The cause of placental abruption is unknown in most cases, although severe direct abdominal trauma, sudden uterine decompression following membrane rupture in polyhydramnios, and vigorous attempts at external cephalic version can all cause placental separation. Pregnancies complicated by prolonged premature rupture of the membranes, chorioamnionitis, pre-eclampsia and fetal growth restriction are at increased risk of placental abruption, and there are associations with increased maternal age and parity, cigarette smoking, cocaine abuse, thrombophilia, raised serum alphafetoprotein, poverty and malnutrition.[14]

The classical clinical presentation of placental abruption is vaginal bleeding and uterine pain, tenderness and contractions. Backache is often a presenting complaint when the placenta is posterior. Bleeding occurs due to separation of the placenta from the underlying decidua either at the edge or in the central area of the placenta. Bleeding into the myometrium may cause sustained contraction, and the uterus may be tense, hard and woody in consistency. Fetal parts may be difficult to palpate. Fetal asphyxia may occur depending on the extent of placental separation and increased uterine tone, which may restrict the uteroplacental circulation, so there may be fetal heart rate abnormalities or absent fetal heart sounds.

The woman may appear pale and shocked although the amount of vaginal bleeding may be slight or even absent despite major bleeding into the uterine muscle or amniotic cavity – 'concealed haemorrhage'. This is different from placenta praevia where most of the bleeding passes quickly into the vagina and is revealed externally. Disseminated intravascular coagulation (DIC) may occur (see Chapter 5). Placental abruption may be divided into grades (Table 4.3).

The clinical presentation of placental abruption varies, and may be difficult to distinguish from preterm labour, placenta praevia or, if vaginal bleeding is absent, from other causes of severe abdominal pain in pregnancy such as uterine rupture, rectus sheath haematoma, red degeneration in a fibroid, torsion or rupture of an ovarian cyst, or appendicitis. Ultrasound will help to rule out some of these conditions, demonstrate the placental site, allow assessment of fetal wellbeing, and may show retroplacental clot. Fresh clot may not be distinguishable from

Table 4.3 Grades of placental abruption[26]	
Grade I	Not recognised clinically before delivery Usually diagnosed by presence of retroplacental clot
Grade II	Intermediate: classical signs of abruption present Fetus is alive
Grade III	Severe: Fetus is dead IIIa: without coagulopathy IIIb: with coagulopathy

placenta on ultrasound but the placenta may appear extremely thick. Cardiotocography should be commenced to assess fetal heart rate patterns and may also show raised baseline uterine tone with superimposed small contractions. Management options in placental abruption include:

- expectant management
- immediate delivery
- management of complications.

If the gestation is less than 37 weeks and the diagnosis uncertain or the degree of abruption minor, conservative management is an option. Careful monitoring of the mother and fetus are important in the early stages. In the longer term, fetal growth and wellbeing should be monitored by serial ultrasound and Doppler and induction of labour should be considered before term, or earlier if there is concern about fetal wellbeing.

If there is significant placental abruption, appropriate resuscitation and maternal and fetal monitoring should be commenced immediately and the fetus delivered as quickly as possible by caesarean section (unless vaginal delivery is imminent). Delay increases the risk of serious maternal complications such as coagulopathy and the risk to the fetus of asphyxia, death or neonatal hypoxic ischaemic encephalopathy. If the fetus is already dead, vaginal delivery is the aim. Rupture of the forewaters may be performed to initiate or accelerate labour. Intravenous oxytocin may be used to encourage contractions but overstimulation should be avoided as there is a risk of uterine rupture. It may be necessary to deliver a dead fetus by caesarean section if attempts at vaginal delivery fail or if bleeding is otherwise uncontrollable.

Other complications include acute renal failure, fetomaternal haemorrhage (which can cause sensitisation in rhesus negative women) and postpartum haemorrhage due to poor uterine contraction following severe bleeding into the myometrium. Perinatal outcome depends on the underlying cause, associated risk factors and degree of fetal asphyxia. The risk of recurrent haemorrhage in subsequent pregnancies is 8–17% after one episode and 25% after two; fetal death due to abruption will recur in 7% of cases; and 30% of all future pregnancies following an abruption will not produce a living child.[14] Maternal mortality may occur, either directly due to haemorrhage – three such deaths were reported to the 2000–2002 CEMD[2] – or due to subsequent complications.

Primary postpartum haemorrhage

Primary postpartum haemorrhage is blood loss of 500 ml or more occurring within 24 hours of delivery. It is usually unpredictable but risk factors include maternal obesity, big baby, increased maternal age, antepartum haemorrhage, previous postpartum haemorrhage, prolonged labour, placenta praevia, operative delivery and emergency caesarean section. The main causes are:

- uterine atony (in about 90% of cases)
- genital tract trauma
- partially retained placenta
- placenta praevia and accreta
- coagulation disorders.

Ten women died in the triennium 2000–2002 as a direct result of postpartum haemorrhage, a significant increase on the previous triennium.[2] Five other women had complications in which significant haemorrhage occurred.

Uterine atony

The most common cause of primary postpartum haemorrhage is uterine atony. It may be due to parity, uterine over-distension during pregnancy, as in multiple pregnancy or polyhydramnios, or retained products.

The first step is to 'rub up' a contraction, then check that the bladder is not distended, then give oxytocics and then if necessary commence appropriate resuscitation. A slow intravenous or intramuscular bolus of ergometrine 500 micrograms or 1 ampoule of Syntometrine® (Alliance, Chippenham, Wilts.), unless contraindicated, may be given and an intravenous infusion of oxytocin, 40 units in 1 litre of Hartmann's solution at 150–250 ml/hour, commenced. Carboprost 250 micrograms may be given intramuscularly to stimulate myometrial contraction (it is not licensed for intramyometrial use). This dose may be repeated after 90 minutes (or sooner, but not earlier than after a 15 minute interval). The total dose should not exceed 2 mg. Carboprost causes increased heart rate, blood pressure, cardiac output and pulmonary vascular resistance and should be used cautiously in women with pre-eclampsia, cardiac problems or asthma.

The placenta and membranes should be delivered and carefully checked for completeness. Ultrasound scan of the uterus may be performed if retained products are suspected; if present, the uterine cavity must be explored under regional or general anaesthesia. The lower genital tract should also be carefully inspected with good exposure and good light for tears or haematoma.

Uterine inversion

Uterine inversion is relatively rare but may cause life-threatening haemorrhage. It may be recognised by failure to palpate the fundus in the abdomen and presence of a vaginal mass (the inverted uterus), which should be replaced without delay by manual or hydrostatic pressure under suitable analgesia or anaesthesia. If this fails, laparotomy may be necessary.

Uterine rupture

Uterine rupture should be suspected in any woman with a previous caesarean or other uterine scar who collapses or develops hypovolaemic shock during pregnancy, during labour or after delivery. It may present with constant lower abdominal pain, cessation of contractions and fetal heart disturbance in the undelivered woman, and vaginal bleeding, which may be slight. If the woman is delivered, the uterine scar may be gently palpated internally (under suitable analgesia or anaesthesia) for signs of rupture; laparotomy may be necessary.

Secondary postpartum haemorrhage

Secondary or 'late' postpartum haemorrhage is any excessive blood loss after the first 24 hours and within 6 weeks of delivery. It is usually due to retained, often infected, products of conception. Occasionally bleeding may occur from a caesarean section incision or vessels in the placental bed, or be due to hydatidiform mole or choriocarcinoma. A vaginal swab should be taken for culture and the woman treated with antibiotics effective against aerobic and anaerobic organisms. Ultrasound scan should be performed. If retained products are present, evacuation of the uterus under general anaesthesia should be done with great care to avoid perforation as the uterus may be soft, especially if infected. If there is clinical evidence of sepsis – pyrexia, tender uterus, offensive discharge – antibiotics should be given intravenously and, if the woman's condition allows, evacuation delayed for 12–24 hours to reduce the risk of septicaemia. Secondary postpartum haemorrhage is not usually massive, but if necessary appropriate resuscitation should be instituted.

Emergency management of major haemorrhage

The signs and symptoms of haemorrhage include a rising pulse rate, falling blood pressure, pallor, sweating, restlessness and oliguria. External bleeding does not always reflect the true extent of blood loss and tachycardia is an important early warning sign.

The immediate management of haemorrhage is the same irrespective of the cause or amount of blood loss. The circulating blood volume must be restored and the bleeding source identified and dealt with promptly, before coagulopathy, hypovolaemic shock and irreversible organ failure develop.

- Establish venous access (minimum two large bore 14 gauge cannulae).
- Take blood for haemoglobin, urea and electrolytes, coagulation screen and cross-matching.
- Order at least 6 units of packed red cells.
- Inform blood transfusion laboratory staff, porters and consultant haematologist immediately of the likely urgent need for large quantities of blood and blood products.
- Inform senior obstetric, midwifery and anaesthetic staff immediately – expert help should be always be sought early.

Fluid replacement should be commenced with a crystalloid such as Hartmann's solution. If blood is not available after 2 litres of crystalloid have been infused, a colloid such as gelatin or pentastarch may be commenced. Fully crossmatched blood is best but in dire circumstances type-specific ABO compatible or uncrossmatched O rhesus negative blood may be given. Blood should be transfused through a blood filter and a blood warmer should be used.

DIC (see Chapter 5) is sometimes part of the presenting condition, for example in placental abruption. Dilutional coagulopathy is often an additional problem when large amounts of fluid are being transfused. Coagulopathy is manifested by prolonged bleeding time and poor clot formation, which contributes significantly to blood loss and frustrates attempts to obtain haemostasis. If coagulopathy is suspected, at least 2 units of fresh frozen plasma, which contains all the clotting factors, should be transfused, with additional plasma and/or cryoprecipitate as guided by coagulation studies, which should be done frequently.

Vital signs should be monitored at frequent intervals dictated by the patient's condition; oxygen may be given; an indwelling bladder catheter should be inserted to measure urine output hourly; central venous and arterial access may be needed; and accurate records of fluid input and output and any drugs given should be kept.

As soon as resuscitation is under way, the bleeding source should be identified and dealt with, the method depending on the specific cause. The immediate management of postpartum uterine atony has been outlined above. Ideally, the woman should be adequately resuscitated and coagulopathy corrected before embarking on surgical procedures but this may not be possible in some circumstances and delaying surgery may be fatal. Post-delivery, interim measures such as bimanual compression of the uterus and compression of the aorta against the sacral promontory are useful temporary measures which may help to control bleeding while waiting for drugs to act or while preparing for laparotomy. If the abdomen is already open, pressure using large packs may temporarily staunch bleeding until more definitive measures can be taken, and may also buy

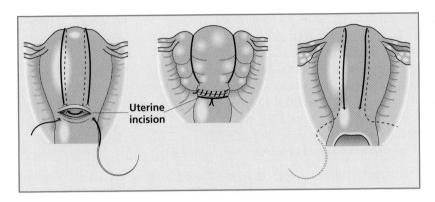

Figure 4.1 The B-Lynch brace suture

time to correct hypovolaemia and coagulopathy with beneficial effects on haemostasis. A non-pneumatic antishock garment, which applies counter-pressure to the lower body, may be useful in situations where blood transfusion is not readily available.[15]

Various surgical techniques designed to control uterine haemorrhage due to atony or rupture without resorting to hysterectomy have been described. Figure-of-eight sutures may be placed directly to control excessive bleeding from the placental bed at caesarean section. The B-Lynch technique[16] may control haemorrhage from the atonic uterus which has failed to respond to medical therapy. The uterus is compressed by a belt and braces type of suture (Figure 4.1).

Uterine packing under adequate analgesia or anaesthesia may be useful where bleeding is due to atony or from a lower segment placental bed.[17] The uterus and vagina are tightly packed, starting from the fundus, with gauze strips tied together, dry or soaked in cold or hot saline or povidone-iodine. Oxytocics should be used, broad spectrum antibiotic cover given, and an indwelling catheter left in the bladder. If successful, the pack is removed in theatre after 24–36 hours. Alternatively, a hydrostatic balloon type catheter, such as a Sengstaken–Blakemore tube or a Rusch urological balloon catheter, may be inserted into the uterus and filled with water or saline.[18] This method has been used successfully in combination with the B-Lynch suture to treat postpartum haemorrhage due to atonic uterus.[19]

Ligation of the uterine arteries, bilateral mass ligation of the uterine vessels,[20] stepwise uterine devascularisation,[21] and bilateral internal iliac or hypogastric artery ligation[22] may all be successful in controlling haemorrhage and preventing hysterectomy but at risk of operative damage to other pelvic vessels and ureters. Only an experienced surgeon, preferably a vascular surgeon, should attempt these procedures.

Figure 4.2   Guidelines for the management of massive obstetric haemorrhage

Call for help

1 Summon most experienced resident staff: obstetrician, anaesthetist and senior midwife.
2 Alert porters, blood transfusion laboratory staff and duty haematologist.
3 Inform consultant obstetrician, consultant anaesthetist and consultant haematologist.
4 Inform duty paediatric registrar and duty paediatric consultant if woman is undelivered.
5 Prepare theatre.

Restore circulating blood volume

1 Elevate foot of bed; if pregnant, position with left lateral tilt. Give oxygen 8 l/minute by face mask.
2 Put in at least two large-bore (14-gauge) peripheral intravenous lines.
3 Take 20–25 ml of blood for crossmatching, FBP, U&E and coagulation screen.
4 Give the following fluids as appropriate: (use fluid warmer and pressure infusion)
   • Hartmann's solution rapid infusion of 2 litres, followed by colloid (gelatin or pentastarch) up to 1.5 litres
   • Transfuse crossmatched blood as soon as available (use blood filter – change every 4 units)
   • If no crossmatched blood and blood is essential, give type-specific blood
   • Uncrossmatched O Rh negative blood should only be used as a last resort.

Correct coagulopathy

1 Give fresh frozen plasma as guided by coagulation screen.
2 Check coagulation screen at intervals.
3 If the platelet count is less than 50×10^9/l, give platelet concentrates.
4 If severe bleeding continues and fibrinogen is less than 1.0 g/dl, give cryoprecipitate.
5 Correct coagulopathy before embarking on major surgery.

(continues on following page)

Monitor

1 Insert a self-retaining urinary catheter to monitor hourly urinary output.
2 Consider insertion of central venous pressure line to monitor fluid replacement (anaesthetist).
3 Consider insertion of arterial line to monitor arterial pressure and blood gases (anaesthetist).
4 Assign one midwife to observations and record keeping:
   - pulse
   - blood pressure (DINAMAP/arterial BP)
   - maternal heart rate (ECG)
   - maternal oxygen concentration (pulse oximeter)
   - central venous pressure
   - urine output (hourly)
   - amount and type of fluids the patient has received
   - amount and type of drugs the patient has received.

Stop the bleeding

1 Antepartum – deliver, usually by caesarean section if fetus alive and coagulation normal.
2 Postpartum – rub up a contraction.
3 Give Syntometrine (ergometrine maleate 500 micrograms, oxytocin 5 units/ml) 1 ampoule or oxytocin 5–10 units intramuscularly or by slow intravenous injection.
4 Set up iv infusion of 40 units of Syntocinon in 1 litre Hartmann's solution at 150–250 ml/hour.
5 Under appropriate anaesthesia, exclude damage to genital tract and retained placental tissue.

If massive haemorrhage continues

1 Consultant obstetrician and consultant anaesthetist should be present.
2 Commence bimanual compression of the uterus.
3 Carboprost 250 micrograms by deep intramuscular injection – may repeat after 90 minutes (minimum interval between doses 15 minutes; maximum 8 doses; beware cardiovascular side effects).
4 The following surgical or interventional procedures may be appropriate:
   - uterine packing or balloon tamponade
   - B-Lynch suture
   - ligation of uterine arteries, internal iliac arteries and ovarian arteries (vascular surgeon)
   - arterial embolisation only if resources and experience available (radiologist)
   - hysterectomy

Selective angiographic arterial embolisation via the femoral artery has also been used to control postpartum haemorrhage.[23] This is a promising technique but its use is limited by the need to have an interventional radiologist and specific equipment readily available, and there can be significant complications such as infection and vessel perforation.

The techniques described above may, if used appropriately, avoid hysterectomy in some cases. Nevertheless, hysterectomy is the definitive treatment for persistent uncontrollable uterine bleeding. The decision, which should be made by a consultant, should not be delayed as prompt action may be lifesaving. Subtotal hysterectomy may be quicker and safer than total hysterectomy.

Minimising risk

Preventive measures for all pregnant women are important, such as checking for and treating anaemia during pregnancy, detection of placenta praevia by ultrasound scan, and active management of the third stage of labour by using prophylactic oxytocics to aid uterine contraction and delivery of the placenta by controlled cord traction.

Haemorrhage can occur suddenly and unexpectedly in any woman. However, some women are at increased risk of bleeding. It is important to identify them antenatally and be prepared for problems. Delivery should take place in a consultant obstetric unit with ready access to a blood bank. Consultant obstetricians and anaesthetists should be directly involved in their care. Staff should be familiar with the emergency management of massive haemorrhage and all obstetric units should have readily available written guidelines – an example is shown in Figure 4.2.

Some women, particularly Jehovah's witnesses, are at risk because their religious or personal beliefs do not allow transfusion of blood or blood products. These women should be identified as early as possible in pregnancy. Documented discussion should take place to ensure that they are fully informed about the risks of refusing blood transfusion in the potential event of life-threatening haemorrhage and to establish their precise wishes if this should occur. Every effort should be made to identify other risk factors for haemorrhage, to avoid the occurrence of haemorrhage and to minimise its effects. Specific recommendations for the management of women who decline blood transfusion even for life-threatening haemorrhage are given in the *Report on Confidential Enquiries into Maternal Deaths in the United Kingdom 2000–2002*.[24] Many hospitals have their own guidelines and specific operation consent forms for Jehovah's witnesses and often have a Jehovah's Witnesses Hospital Liaison Committee who may be involved in discussions with these women.

Training issues

Shorter working hours and the relative rarity of life-threatening haemorrhage mean that trainee obstetricians may be unfamiliar with massive haemorrhage and may not appreciate the speed at which acute torrential bleeding can develop into circulatory collapse, exsanguination and irreversible shock. In other situations, concealed or persistent bleeding may go unrecognised until the patient suddenly decompensates and develops hypovolaemic shock. There is often a short but critical window of opportunity where prompt and effective action may make the difference between life and death. Failure to recognise the gravity of the situation, to commence appropriate and adequate resuscitative measures, and to involve senior staff at an early stage are recurrent themes in the CEMD.

Training programmes need to address these issues with targeted teaching, mandatory attendance at emergency training courses such as Advanced Life Support in Obstetrics and Management of Obstetric Emergencies and Trauma. Induction programmes for junior doctors in

---

Key points

- Massive haemorrhage is a major cause of maternal mortality.
- Haemorrhage is often the cause of death associated with ectopic pregnancy, which may present atypically. A high index of suspicion of ectopic pregnancy should be maintained and pregnancy testing performed if there is any doubt.
- A senior obstetrician should always perform caesarean section for placenta praevia.
- The immediate management of primary postpartum haemorrhage due to uterine atony is to 'rub up a contraction' and give an oxytocic drug.
- Expert senior help (consultant obstetrician, anaesthetist and haematologist, and senior midwife) should be called early in cases of major haemorrhage.
- Good communication between all staff, including blood transfusion laboratory and porters, is essential.
- Prompt institution of resuscitation and definitive steps to stop bleeding are important, as delay can be fatal.
- Anticipation and prevention of potential problems is important.
- Regular staff training sessions and practice emergency drills improve the management of real emergencies.

---

obstetrics should include a session on recognising and dealing with major haemorrhage. Written information containing guidelines for management of haemorrhage (Figure 4.2) and contact details of important personnel should be provided. Anticipating problems and calling senior medical staff at an early stage should be encouraged.

Multidisciplinary practical emergency training drills should be held regularly. Debriefing following these drills and real situations provides opportunity to streamline procedures, improve communications and highlight training needs.

References

1   Drife J. Management of primary postpartum haemorrhage. *Br J Obstet Gynaecol* 1997;104:275–7.

2   Hall MH. Haemorrhage. In: Lewis G, editor. *Why Mothers Die 2000–2002. The Sixth Report of the Confidential Enquiries into Maternal Deaths in the United Kingdom.* London: RCOG Press; 2004. p. 81–8.

3   Waterstone M, Bewley S, Wolfe C. Incidence and predictors of severe obstetric morbidity: case control study. *BMJ* 2001;322:1089–93.

4   Jouppila P. Postpartum haemorrhage. *Curr Opin Obstet Gynecol* 1995;7:446–50.

5   Walker ID, Walker JJ, Colvin BT, Letsky EA, Rivers R, Stevens R. Investigation and management of haematological disorders in pregnancy. *J Clin Pathol* 1994;47:100–108.

6   Bonnar J. Massive Obstetric Haemorrhage. In: Thompson W, TambyRaja RL, editors. *Emergencies in Obstetrics and Gynaecology.* London: Baillière-Tindall; 2000. p. 1–18.

7   Neilson JP. Early Pregnancy Deaths. In: Lewis G, editor. *Why Mothers Die 2000–2002. The Sixth Report of the Confidential Enquiries into Maternal Deaths in the United Kingdom.* London: RCOG Press; 2004. p. 102–8.

8   Rajkhowa M, Glass MR, Rutherford AJ, Balen AH, Sharma V, Cuckle HS. Trends in the incidence of ectopic pregnancy in England and Wales from 1966 to 1996. *Br J Obstet Gynaecol* 2000;107:369–74.

9   Royal College of Obstetricians and Gynaecologists. *The Management of Tubal Pregnancies.* Guideline No. 21. London: RCOG; 1999.

10 Drife J. Bleeding in pregnancy. In: Chamberlain G, Steer P, editors. *Turnbull's Obstetrics.* 3rd ed. Churchill Livingstone; 2001. p. 211–28.

11 Royal College of Obstetricians and Gynaecologists. *Placenta Praevia: Diagnosis and Management.* Guideline No. 27. London: RCOG; 2001.

12 Dawson WB, Dumas MD, Romano WM, Gagnon R, Gratton RJ, Mowbray RD. Translabial ultrasonography and placenta previa: does measurement of the os-placental distance predict outcome? *J Ultrasound Med* 1996;15:441–6.

13 Clark SL, Koonings PP, Phelan JP. Placenta praevia/accreta and prior caesarean section. *Obstet Gynecol* 1985;66:89–92.

14 Konje JC, Taylor DJ. Bleeding in late pregnancy. In: James DJ, Steer PJ, Weiner CP, Gonik B, editors. *High Risk Pregnancy.* 2nd ed. London: WB Saunders; 1999. p. 111–28.

15 Hensleigh PA. Anti-shock garment provides resuscitation and haemostasis for obstetric haemorrhage. *BJOG* 2002;109:1377–84.

16 B-Lynch C, Coker A, Lawal AH, Abu J, Cowen MJ. The B-Lynch surgical technique for the control of massive postpartum haemorrhage: an alternative to hysterectomy? Five cases reported. *Br J Obstet Gynaecol* 1997;104:372–75.

17 Maier RC. Control of postpartum haemorrhage with uterine packing. *Am J Obstet Gynecol* 1993;169:317–23.

18 Johanson R, Kumar M, Obhrai M, Young P. Management of massive postpartum haemorrhage: use of a hydrostatic balloon to avoid laparotomy. *BJOG* 2001;108:420–22.

19 Danso D, Reginald P. Combined B-Lynch suture with intrauterine balloon catheter triumphs over massive postpartum haemorrhage. *BJOG* 2002;109:963.

20 O'Leary JA. Uterine artery ligation in the control of postcaesarean haemorrhage. *J Reprod Med* 1995;40:189–93.

21 AbdRabbo SA. Stepwise uterine devascularisation: A novel technique for management of uncontrollable postpartum haemorrhage with preservation of the uterus. *Am J Obstet Gynecol* 1994;171:694–700.

22 Gilstrap LC, Ramin SM. Postpartum haemorrhage. *Clin Obstet Gynecol* 1994;37:824–30.

23 Hansch E, Chitkara U, McAlpine J, El-Sayed Y, Daka MD, Razavi MK. Pelvic arterial embolization for control of obstetric haemorrhage: a five year experience.*Am J Obstet Gynecol* 1999;180:1454–60.

24 Hall MH. Haemorrhage. Guidelines for the management and treatment of obstetric haemorrhage in women who decline blood transfusion. In: Lewis G, editor. *Why Mothers Die 2000–2002. Sixth Report of the Confidential Enquiries into Maternal Deaths in the United Kingdom*. London: RCOG Press; 2004. p 94–5.

25 Mascarenhas L. Review No. 97/07 Ectopic Pregnancy. In: *Personal Assessment in Continuing Education Reviews and Answers Volume 2*. London: RCOG; 1999. p. 76–82.

26 Sher G, Statland BE. Abruptio placentae with coagulopathy: a rational basis for management. *Clin Obstet Gynecol* 1985;28:15–23.

5 Disseminated intravascular coagulation

Disseminated intravascular coagulation (DIC) is not a disease or a symptom. It is a syndrome, characterised by a dynamic process of intravascular coagulation disseminated throughout the microcirculation resulting in thrombin generation and intravascular fibrin formation. Massive continuing activation of coagulation results in consumption of clotting factors and platelets. Thrombin generation is compounded by simultaneous depression of the natural anticoagulant mechanisms such as antithrombin and the thrombomodulin/protein C/protein S system. The process may be accompanied by secondary fibrinolysis or inhibition of fibrinolysis due to high circulating levels of plasminogen activator inhibitor-1.

DIC is an acquired disorder secondary to underlying pathology including a variety of obstetric complications. The clinical presentation is due to microthrombi generated in the microcirculation and consequent organ failure and/or a bleeding diathesis. There is no single test for DIC. Diagnosis depends on an awareness of the conditions which may be complicated by DIC combined with a variety of laboratory tests. The cornerstone of management of DIC is treatment of the underlying disorder.

Fibrin formation results from activation of the coagulation cascade. Normally, tissue factor, the physiological trigger for coagulation activation, is separated from the circulating blood by the endothelial cell barrier but, when this is disrupted by injury, tissue factor can bind with factors VII and VIIa, initiating coagulation via the extrinsic coagulation cascade and resulting in thrombin generation. The generation and activity of thrombin are tightly regulated by multiple natural anticoagulant pathways including antithrombin, thrombomodulin/protein C/protein S and tissue factor pathway inhibitor. Thrombin generation with subsequent fibrin formation is normally localised to the site of injury.

Pathogenesis

DIC is characterised by an imbalance between prothrombotic and antithrombotic activities. It may complicate a wide range of clinical disorders, including tissue destruction associated with surgery or trauma, serious bacterial or nonbacterial infection, malignancy and a variety of obstetric mishaps. Within the past 5 years, the mechanisms involved in the pathogenesis of DIC have become clearer. Much of the information has been gleaned from observations on patients with sepsis or from experimental sepsis models.

Activation of the extrinsic coagulation (tissue factor/factor VIIa) pathway appears to be the primary activating path in sepsis induced DIC. Inhibition of the tissue factor/factor VIIa pathway with specific monoclonal antibodies results in inhibition of thrombin generation in endotoxin challenged chimpanzees.[1] In healthy humans given a bolus injection of endotoxin, the administration of tissue factor pathway inhibitor produces a dose-dependent inhibition of the activation of coagulation.[2] Activation of the extrinsic coagulation cascade follows endothelial damage and enhanced expression and release of tissue factor. Increased expression and release of tissue factor may be a direct action of specific microorganism cell components (membrane lipopolysaccharides or endotoxins) or it may be mediated via activation of cytokines such as tumour necrosis factor alpha and interleukin-6.

Experiments in human endotoxaemia and in humans infused with endotoxin induced mediator tissue necrosis factors demonstrate that the intrinsic (contact) coagulation cascade is not activated.[3] However, endotoxaemia may activate factor XII leading to the conversion of prekallikrein to kallikrein and kininogens to kinins which can mediate increased vascular permeability, vasodilation and shock. In experimental models inhibition of the intrinsic coagulation path ameliorates hypotension but not DIC.[4]

Increased consumption/degradation and reduced production result in low levels of the most important natural inhibitor of thrombin, antithrombin. Additionally, significant depression of the thrombo-modulin/protein C/protein S system may occur in DIC. Reduced protein C activity due to downregulation of thrombomodulin has been demonstrated.[5] Experimental bacteraemia and endotoxaemia result in an immediate increase in fibrinolytic activity probably owing to the release of plasminogen activators from the endothelium. This profibrinolytic response is however rapidly followed by a sustained suppression of fibrinolytic activity due to increased release of plasminogen activator inhibitor 1.

Whatever the underlying pathology, in DIC, activation of the extrinsic coagulation cascade follows increased release or expression of tissue factor. When the natural anticoagulant pathways are overwhelmed by massive pathologic activation of coagulation, thrombin activity is no longer contained and circulating thrombin causes widespread fibrin formation with histologically visible microthrombi and thrombotic obstruction of small and middle-sized vessels. Red blood cell fragmentation is evident on

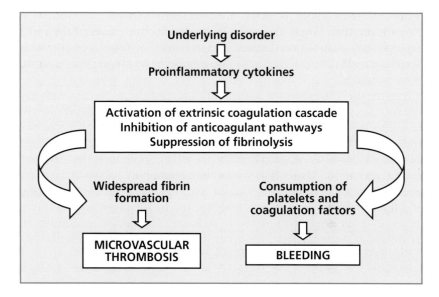

Figure 5.1 Pathogenesis of disseminated intravascular coagulation

peripheral blood films – thrombotic microangiopathy – and blood flow to end organs is compromised with resultant organ dysfunction.[6] Suppression of fibrinolytic activity further increases the thrombotic tendency. Continuing consumption of coagulation factors and platelets causes an increased bleeding risk (Figure 5.1).

Clinical presentation

The clinical presentation of DIC is variable. Sometimes there is little obvious apart from oozing from venepuncture sites but some patients present with serious bleeding. On other occasions the presentation is primarily thrombotic with manifest thromboembolic disease or with clinically less apparent microvascular disease presenting as organ dysfunction.

CHRONIC COMPENSATED DIC

If the activation of coagulation is slow, provided that the liver can compensate for the consumption of clotting factors and the bone marrow maintains an adequate platelet count, severe bleeding is unlikely. Occasionally, patients may have minor skin or mucosal bleeding. Women with chronic compensated DIC may be asymptomatic or may have manifestations of venous or arterial thrombosis.

ACUTE DECOMPENSATED DIC

If the initiating event is more dramatic with explosive activation of coagulation, the clinical picture is dominated by the effects of the rapid depletion of coagulation factors and platelets. Patients present with petechiae and bruising. Frequently also there is oozing from venepuncture sites, wound sites and mucosal surfaces. The bleeding may become life-threatening if it involves the gastrointestinal tract, lungs, central nervous system, the placental bed or operative sites. Acute renal failure due to microthrombosis of afferent arterioles resulting in cortical ischaemia and/or acute tubular necrosis secondary to hypotension or sepsis develops in around 25–40% of people with acute DIC. Jaundice due to liver dysfunction and to haemolysis is common. Pulmonary haemorrhage with haemoptysis and dyspnoea may result from vascular endothelial damage, and diffuse pulmonary microthrombosis due to DIC augments the lung injury of adult respiratory distress syndrome. In addition a number of neurological abnormalities may occur in people with DIC. These include coma, delirium and transient focal neurological signs.

Disseminated intravascular coagulation in obstetrics

Obstetric complications are frequently associated with clinically severe DIC (Table 5.1). Several obstetric complications such as placental abruption, amniotic fluid embolism and septic abortion are associated with acute decompensated DIC, while others such as pre-eclampsia, the HELLP syndrome (haemolysis, elevated liver enzymes, and low platelet count) and retained dead fetus may cause a more chronic low-grade compensated DIC.

PLACENTAL ABRUPTION

Placental abruption (see Chapter 4) means the premature separation of a normally implanted placenta after 20 weeks of gestation. Usually,

Table 5.1 Obstetric complications predisposing to acute or chronic DIC

Acute	Chronic
Amniotic fluid embolism	Pre-eclampsia
Placental abruption	HELLP syndrome
Septic abortion	Retained dead fetus
Acute fatty liver	
Uterine rupture	
Septicaemia	
Extensive surgery	

abruption is the result of rupture of maternal vessels in the decidua basalis but, rarely, the bleeding can originate from fetal placental vessels. The amount of bleeding does not correlate with the extent of maternal haemorrhage and cannot be used as a predictor of the severity of the problem. DIC occurs in around 10–20% of cases of severe abruption. DIC probably results from infusion of tissue factor and/or other thromboplastic material from the disrupted decidua and damaged placental bed into the maternal circulation.

AMNIOTIC FLUID EMBOLISM

Amniotic fluid embolism is a catastrophic condition which occurs during pregnancy or shortly after delivery. The maternal mortality rate is around 60–90% and survivors may suffer severe neurological damage.[7] The onset of symptoms most commonly occurs during labour or immediately after delivery. The major signs include hypoxia, respiratory failure and cardiogenic shock. In addition about 40% of patients develop DIC. Haemorrhage as a result of DIC may occur coincidentally with the initial cardiopulmonary symptoms, may follow these symptoms or in some cases may be the presenting feature.

SEPTIC ABORTION

Overt DIC occurs in 30–50% of women with Gram-negative sepsis but DIC may also occur in association with Gram-positive sepsis and in nonbacterial infections.

TRAUMA OR EXTENSIVE SURGERY

Release of tissue enzymes and/or phospholipids from damaged tissues into the systemic circulation triggers activation of cytokine networks and the haemostatic system.

PRE-ECLAMPSIA AND THE HELLP SYNDROME

Pre-eclampsia is characterised by the development of hypertension and proteinuria in the second half of pregnancy. Maternal endothelial activation due to widespread cytokine mediated oxidative stress and inflammation causes the endothelial surface to change from antithrombotic to prothrombotic.[8] Coagulation is activated and plasminogen activator inhibitor-1 levels increase. Abnormalities of the global coagulation screening tests are unusual but more subtle evidence of coagulation activation such as elevated thrombin antithrombin complex levels is usually demonstrable. Ninety percent of patients have reduced levels of protein C and antithrombin and 40% have elevated D-dimer levels. Platelet activation also occurs and thrombocytopenia occurs in about one-quarter of women with pre-eclampsia. Acute decompensated DIC is rare in the absence of placental abruption. The fall in antithrombin levels seen in pre-eclampsia is not seen in thrombotic thrombocytopenic purpura[9] and thus may be diagnostically useful.

Four to twelve percent of women with pre-eclampsia meet the diagnostic criteria for HELLP:

- microangiopathic haemolysis
- elevated liver enzymes (SGOT >70 iu/l, LDH >600 iu/l, bilirubin >1.2 mg/dl)
- low platelets (<100 x 10^9/l);

but thrombocytopenia and abnormal liver function tests can also occur in the absence of significant hypertension and proteinuria. The majority of cases present late in pregnancy but HELLP may present postpartum, usually within 48 hours of delivery. The clinical presentation varies. Most patients complain of abdominal pain and tenderness and some have nausea and vomiting. A few present with pulmonary oedema or ascites. Clinical evidence of impaired coagulation is unusual at presentation although the platelet count may be < 50 x 10^9/l. Signs of DIC occur in about 20% of patients.[10] Acute renal failure may develop in those with DIC.

Thrombotic microangiopathies comprise a group of disorders, including thrombotic thrombocytopenic purpura and haemolytic uraemic syndrome, which are the result of platelet activation. Although some characteristics of thrombotic microangiopathies may mimic the clinical picture of DIC, they are a separate group of disorders beyond the scope of this chapter. The distinction between these disorders and pre-eclampsia and HELLP is,

Table 5.2 Presenting features of pre-eclampsia, HELLP, TTP, HUS and DIC

Diagnosis	DIC	Pre-eclampsia	HELLP	TTP	HUS
Onset	Any time	>34 weeks	>34 weeks	<24 weeks	Postpartum
Hypertension	-	+++	+/-	rare	+/-
CNS signs	+/-	+/-	+/-	+++	+/-
Liver signs	+/-	+/-	+++	+/-	+/-
Renal signs	+/-	+	+	+/-	+++
Fever	+/-	-	-	+/-	-/+
Haemolysis	+	+	++	+++	++
Platelets ↓	+++	+/-	++	+++	++
Coagulopathy	+++	+/-	+/-	-	-

DIC = disseminated intravascular coagulation; HELLP = haemolysis, elevated liver enzymes and low platelets syndrome; TTP = thrombotic thrombocytopenic purpura; HUS = haemolytic uraemic syndrome

HAEMORRHAGE AND THROMBOSIS FOR THE MRCOG AND BEYOND

however, important for therapeutic and prognostic reasons. Pre-eclampsia and HELLP are associated with thrombocytopenia and in severe cases with DIC there may also be prolongation of the activated partial thromboplastin time (APTT) and prothrombin time (PT). The spectrum of clinical and laboratory features which may help distinguish these conditions is summarised in Table 5.2. Antithrombin levels fall in pre-eclampsia and HELLP. Thrombocytopenic purpura and haemolytic uraemic syndrome are associated with isolated thrombocytopenia without abnormalities in the global screening tests of coagulation and normal antithrombin levels.

Expeditious delivery of the fetus is the mainstay of therapy in pre-eclampsia and HELLP. Laboratory parameters may deteriorate initially following delivery but improvement within 2–4 days postpartum usually occurs in uncomplicated cases. Delivery has no effect on maternal outcome in women with thrombotic thrombocytopenic purpura.

ACUTE FATTY LIVER OF PREGNANCY

Acute fatty liver of pregnancy is characterised by microvesicular fatty infiltration of hepatocytes without inflammation or necrosis. Affected women usually present in the second half of pregnancy close to term but some present after delivery. Women with acute fatty liver of pregnancy have elevated serum aminotransferase levels but a normal platelet count unless the patient has progressed to DIC. The onset of DIC is marked by a significant reduction in antithrombin levels. The major differential diagnosis is from HELLP syndrome. The treatment of acute fatty liver of pregnancy is delivery after maternal stabilisation.

RETAINED DEAD FETUS

Retained dead fetus syndrome is associated with a slowly developing low grade compensated DIC. Patients may have reduced fibrinogen levels and mild thrombocytopenia. The incidence of haemostatic abnormality increases with the length of time for which the fetus has been retained *in utero* following its death. Serious spontaneous haemorrhage is unusual but bleeding during and after delivery may occur if the deficiencies are not corrected.

Diagnosis

The basis of the diagnosis of DIC is an appreciation of the underlying disorders in which DIC can develop. Because acute DIC requires urgent intervention, DIC must always be considered where a complex coagulation disorder is noted in a woman with an underlying disorder which may be associated with DIC. The diagnosis of acute DIC is suggested by the history and clinical presentation. The woman is usually moderately to severely thrombocytopenic and there is evidence of red blood cell fragmentation on the peripheral blood film. Chronic DIC may be more difficult to diagnose but the clinical history and examination should raise the suspicion and lead to appropriate investigation. Table 5.3 summarises the laboratory findings in women with DIC.

GLOBAL COAGULATION TESTS IN DIC

The standard approach to the diagnosis of DIC has been to rely on the platelet count in conjunction with classic global screening tests of coagulation – APTT, PT and thrombin time (TT). Prolongation of the PT reflects reduced activity of the components of the extrinsic and final common coagulation paths including factors VII, X and V. The APTT measures components of the intrinsic coagulation path and is sensitive to deficiencies of factors XII, XI, IX and VIII. It is less sensitive than the PT to deficiencies in the final common path. These tests are nonspecific but are

Table 5.3 Diagnosis of disseminated intravascular coagulation

Compensated activation of haemostasis (early acute DIC or chronic DIC)

No symptoms	
No measurable consumption of components	PT, APTT, TT: within normal
	Platelet count: within normal
Activation markers increased	F1+2, TAT: elevated
	Soluble fibrin may be increased
Inhibitor levels may be reduced	Antithrombin slightly reduced
Peripheral blood film	Occasional RBC fragments

Decompensated activation of haemostasis (acute DIC)

Increased bleeding and decreased organ function (kidneys, lungs, liver)	
Consumption of coagulation factors	PT and APTT prolonged
	TT normal or prolonged
	Fibrinogen normal or reduced
Consumption of platelets	Platelet count reduced
Activation markers increased	FDPs, F1+2, TAT: elevated
	Soluble fibrin increased
Inhibitor levels reduced	Antithrombin reduced
Peripheral blood film	Frequent RBC fragments

APTT = activated partial thromboplastin time; PT = prothrombin time;
TT = thrombin time; FDP = fibrin degradation product; TAT = thrombin antithrombin complex;
F1+2 = prothrombin fragment 1 + 2; RBC = red blood cell

rapid and simple to perform and useful in the diagnosis of DIC if combined with measurement of fibrinogen and FDP levels. Normal APPT or PT results do not however exclude DIC. Similarly, particularly in pregnant women, the TT and fibrinogen levels may be within normal 'non-pregnant' ranges in some women with DIC. Changes in these global screening tests do not occur at the same rate and repeat testing may be necessary to detect trends.

Isolated thrombocytopenia is not specific for DIC. Since elevation of FDP levels (including D-dimers) may occur in association with a variety of clinical disorders including DIC, deep vein thrombosis and inflammation, elevated FDPs or D-dimers cannot be regarded as a stand-alone tests for DIC. A falling platelet count occurring concurrently with a rising level of FDPs is however a useful indicator of DIC.

Global tests of coagulation are useful in the diagnosis of acute DIC although identifying DIC at an early stage by these means may be difficult especially if repeat testing is not performed. They are of limited value in patients with chronic compensated DIC where little abnormality may be observed in the results of these investigations.

SCORING SYSTEMS IN DIC DIAGNOSIS

In an attempt to standardise the procedure for diagnosing DIC, various scoring systems have been developed. The system developed by the Japanese Ministry of Health and Welfare takes into account both clinical and laboratory data placing particular emphasis on the finding of a low platelet count and raised FDPs.[11] Although these scoring systems may be unwieldy in an emergency situation and unnecessary where there is frank evidence of coagulation activation they may be useful in the diagnosis of early DIC particularly if encompassed within a scheme which ensures structured repeat testing.

MOLECULAR MARKERS IN DIC DIAGNOSIS

Because the global tests of coagulation have limited application in the diagnosis of early or low grade chronic DIC there has been considerable interest in the use of more sensitive molecular markers of haemostasis activation (Figure 5.2). A variety of markers of coagulation or fibrinolytic activation such as thrombin-antithrombin complexes, prothrombin fragment 1 + 2 and soluble fibrin monomers have been shown to be helpful in the diagnosis of DIC including low grade chronic DIC but these tests are rarely available in the emergency setting and frequently unavailable even on a routine basis.

Depletion of naturally occurring anticoagulants such as antithrombin or protein C have been related to clinical outcome and have been the focus

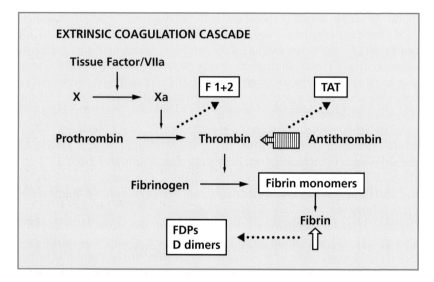

Figure 5.2 Molecular markers of coagulation and fibrinolytic system activation; F1+2 = prothrombin fragment 1 + 2; TAT = thrombin antithrombin complex; FDP = fibrin degradation product

of replacement therapy in clinical trials. However their sensitivity for the diagnosis of early DIC is unclear.

Management

Evidence on which to base guidance on the management of DIC is scant. Acute DIC is a serious complication which carries with it a high risk of mortality. It is generally accepted that the cornerstone of management of DIC is treatment of the underlying cause. In addition supportive therapies based on an understanding of the pathogenesis of DIC may be useful.

PLASMA AND PLATELET THERAPY

Low levels of platelets and of clotting factors may increase the risk of bleeding. Replacement of platelets and/or clotting factors with fresh frozen plasma would seem rational in women who have reduced levels of clotting factors and/or platelets but the efficacy of this therapy has not been proven in randomised controlled trials. Theoretically, replacement therapy may 'add fuel to the fire' but this has not been demonstrated either clinically or in studies.

Plasma and platelet replacement therapy should not be based on laboratory results but offered only to women who are already bleeding or in danger of bleeding – for example at delivery or if an invasive procedure is planned. Concentrates of coagulation factors should be avoided since they are potentially thrombogenic.

ANTICOAGULANTS

The administration of heparin or other anticoagulants to interrupt the coagulopathy in DIC may appear logical. The safety of heparin treatment in women with DIC is however debatable and a beneficial effect on clinical outcome has never been demonstrated in a controlled trial. The administration of heparin or low molecular weight heparin is generally limited to women with low-grade chronic compensated DIC who have predominantly thrombotic manifestations, such as thrombophlebitis or who are at risk of venous thromboembolism.

COAGULATION INHIBITOR CONCENTRATES

A number of controlled trials of antithrombin concentrates have been reported in women with DIC. In most of these trials DIC has been associated with underlying sepsis or septic shock. All of the trials show some benefits in terms of improved laboratory results and shortening of the duration of DIC. Some trials showed a modest reduction in DIC mortality in antithrombin treated women but the effect did not reach statistical significance in individual trials In a meta-analysis of the effect of antithrombin treatment on DIC mortality in six published trials Levi et al.[12] reported a statistically significant reduction in mortality (from 42% to 37%: odds ratio 0.59; 95% CI 0.39–0.87). It is not clear however which women may benefit from antithrombin treatment. In the UK the availability of antithrombin concentrate is at present limited.

Depression of the protein C system significantly contributes to the pathophysiology of DIC in some women. There have been some reports of successful treatment with protein C concentrates in women with DIC[13] but adequately controlled trials have not been performed.

Activated protein C (aPC) has both anticoagulant and anti-inflammatory activities. In a randomised, double-blind trial, 1690 women with severe sepsis received an intravenous infusion of recombinant aPC or placebo for 96 hours. The trial was terminated early because a statistically significant favourable result was observed in the recombinant aPC treated group. The mortality rate was 30.8% in the placebo treated group compared with 24.7% in the group given recombinant aPC.[14]

In view of the pivotal role of tissue factor in the pathogenesis of DIC, administration of recombinant tissue factor pathway inhibitor may prove to be of benefit. In animal studies administration of tissue factor pathway inhibitor significantly reduces fibrin deposition in organs and prevents consumption of clotting factors.[15] Tissue factor pathway inhibitor is under trial in humans with DIC.

ANTIFIBRINOLYTIC AGENTS

The use of antifibrinolytic agents is not generally recommended in women with DIC because fibrin deposition, which is in part due to reduced fibrinolytic activity, is an important feature of DIC.

Key points

- DIC is an acquired disorder secondary to underlying pathology, including obstetric complications such as placental abruption, amniotic fluid embolism, septic abortion, retained dead fetus, pre-eclampsia and HELLP syndrome.
- The clinical presentation is a consequence of microthrombi formation in the microcirculation which is manifested by organ failure and/or a bleeding diathesis.
- In chronic compensated DIC, severe bleeding is unlikely, but in acute situations life-threatening haemorrhage can rapidly occur.
- The diagnosis of DIC is suggested by the clinical history and presentation, together with moderate to severe thrombocytopenia and evidence of red cell fragmentation on the peripheral blood film. Serial coagulation screening is also helpful.
- The cornerstone of management of DIC is treatment of the underlying disorder.
- Plasma and platelet replacement therapy may be given to women who are already bleeding or at high risk of bleeding, for example at delivery.
- Coagulation inhibitor concentrates may have a place in treatment of DIC but antifibrinolytic agents are not recommended.

References

1   Biemond BJ, Levi M, ten Cate H, *et al*. Complete inhibition of endotoxin induced coagulation activation in chimpanzees with a monoclonal antibody to factor VII/VIIa. *Thromb Haemost* 1995;73:223–30.

2   De Jonge E, Dekkers PE, Creasey AA, *et al*. Tissue factor pathway inhibitor dose dependently inhibits coagulation activation without influencing the fibrinolytic and cytokine response during human endotoxaemia. *Blood* 2000;95:1124–9.

3   van der Poll T, Buller HR, ten Cate H, *et al*. Activation of coagulation after administration of tumour necrosis factor to normal subjects. *N Engl J Med* 1990;322:1622–7.

4   Pixley RA, de la Cadena R, Page JD, *et al*. The contact system contributes to hypotension but not disseminated intravascular coagulation in lethal bacteraemia. In vivo use of a monoclonal anti-factor XII antibody to block contact activation in baboons. *J Clin Invest* 1993;91:61–8.

5   Conway EM, Rosenberg RD. Tumour necrosis factor suppresses transcription of the thrombomodulin gene in endothelial cells. *Mol Cell Biol* 1988;8:5588–92.

6   Levi M, ten Cate H. Disseminated intravascular coagulation. *N Engl J Med* 1999;341:586–92.

7   Clark SL, Hankins GD, Dudley DA, *et al*. Amniotic fluid embolism: Analysis of the national registry. *Am J Obstet Gynecol* 1995;172:1158–69.

8   Hunt BJ, Jurd KM. Endothelial cell activation. *BMJ* 1998;316:1328–9.

9   Sagripanti A, Carpi A, Baicchi U, *et al*. Plasmatic parameters of coagulation activation in thrombotic microangiopathy. *Biomed Pharmacother* 1996;50:357–62.

10   Sibai BM, Ramadan MK, Usta I, *et al*. Maternal morbidity and mortality in 442 pregnancies with haemolysis, elevated liver enzymes and low platelets (HELLP syndrome). *Am J Obstet Gynecol* 1993;169:1000–1006.

11   Wada H, Wakita Y, Nakase T, *et al*. Outcome of disseminated intravascular coagulation in relation to the score when treatment was begun. *Thromb Haemost* 1995;74:848–52.

12   Levi M, de Jonge E, van der Poll T, *et al*. Disseminated intravascular coagulation. *Thromb Haemost* 1999;82:695–705.

13   Smith OP, WhiteB, Vaughan D, *et al*. Use of protein C concentrate, heparin and haemodiafiltration in meningococcus-induced purpura fulminans. *Lancet* 1997;350:1590–93.

14   Bernard GR, Vincent JL, Laterre PF, *et al*. Efficacy and safety of recombinant human activated protein C for severe sepsis. *N Engl J Med* 2001;344:699–709.

15   Creasey AA, Chang ACK, Feigen L, *et al*. Tissue factor pathway inhibitor reduces mortality from Escherichia coli septic shock. *J Clin Invest* 1993;91:2850–60.

6 Gynaecological problems in women with bleeding disorders

Excessive or abnormal vaginal bleeding are the most common symptoms when women present to a gynaecologist. The cause is usually gynaecological pathology but occasionally gynaecologists may encounter women with such symptoms secondary to inherited or acquired bleeding disorders. This chapter aims to increase awareness and provide basic information about these relatively uncommon disorders. Gynaecological complications associated with these disorders and their management will also be discussed.

Inherited bleeding disorders

VON WILLEBRAND'S DISORDER

Inherited bleeding disorders in women are far more common than previously suspected. Von Willebrand's disorder seems to be the most common inherited haemorrhagic disorder in women, with an estimated prevalence of 1–3%. Von Willebrand's disorder is a consequence of quantitative and/or qualitative defects of von Willebrand factor (VWF), a protein that is necessary for platelet adhesion and thrombus formation and which also serves as a carrier for factor FVIII.

Von Willebrand's disorder demonstrates extreme clinical and genetic heterogeneity depending on the subtype considered. There are three main types: types 1 and 3 caused by quantitative and type 2 caused by qualitative defects in VWF protein.

- Type 1 (70% of all cases) is the most common form of the disease. It is characterised by low plasma levels, usually between 5 iu/dl and 40 iu/dl, of FVIII (normal range 50–150 iu/dl) and VWF (normal range 50–175 iu/dl). This is caused by reduced production of normally functioning VWF, resulting in a secondary defect of FVIII.
- Type 2 (15–20% of cases) comprises many different subtypes. In most cases, this results in an abnormal multimeric structure of VWF and hence abnormal platelet–VWF–vessel wall interaction.

- Type 3 is the least common of all forms of Von Willebrand's disorder and is characterised by very low levels of plasma VWF and FVIII, with severe bleeding manifestations.

Types 1 and 2 are transmitted as autosomal dominant trait. Type 3 is autosomal recessive in inheritance.

CARRIERSHIP OF HAEMOPHILIA A AND B

The other important inherited bleeding disorders in women are carriership of haemophilia A (FVIII deficiency) and haemophilia B (FIX deficiency). Haemophilias A and B are X-linked disorders. Therefore, the clotting factor level is expected to be around 50% of normal in carriers as they have only one affected chromosome. However, a wide range of values (22–116 iu/dl) has been reported[1] as a result of random inactivation of one of the two X chromosomes, the process called lyonisation.[2] A significant number of haemophilia carriers may have extremely low factor levels due to extreme lyonisation and are therefore at risk of severe bleeding complications.

FACTOR XI DEFICIENCY

Factor XI (FXI) deficiency is a less common bleeding disorder but is particularly prevalent in Ashkenazi Jews. It is one of the most common genetic disorders in this population with a heterozygous frequency of 8%.[3] In the UK, FXI deficiency accounts for 3% of all people with a bleeding disorder. A significant number have no known Jewish ancestry but the exact frequency in non-Jewish people is unknown. FXI deficiency is autosomal in inheritance, with severe deficiency in homozygotes (FXI <15 iu/dl; normal range 70–150 iu/dl) and partial deficiency in heterozygotes.[4] There is poor correlation between FXI level and bleeding tendency in people with FXI deficiency.[4] Some with severe deficiency may not bleed following trauma, while some heterozygotes have excessive bleeding after such a challenge. The bleeding tendency may also vary in the same individual following haemostatic challenge.[3] This is dependent upon genotype, site of surgery and the presence of additional coagulation factor defects, most commonly Von Willebrand's disorder.

RARE INHERITED BLEEDING DISORDERS

These include prothrombin, fibrinogen, FVII, combined FV/FVIII, FX and FXIII deficiencies. Although menorrhagia has been reported, there is limited data and experience with women affected by these disorders. Hereditary platelet function disorders (Glanzmann thrombocythenia, Bernard–Soulier disease and storage pool disease) are rare but recognised causes of menorrhagia. Because of the rarity of these conditions and the need for specialised investigations and treatment, these women need to be managed in units where haematologists experienced in haemophilia care, laboratory facilities for monitoring factor levels, and blood products are readily available.

Acquired bleeding disorders

Immune idiopathic thrombocytopenic purpura (ITP) in adults is usually a chronic disorder with an insidious onset of minor bleeding symptoms. It has not been shown to be an underlying cause of menorrhagia. ITP can also be an acute disorder, with an abrupt onset of bleeding symptoms. This is more common in younger age groups, typically in children less than 10 years old, and has also been reported to be a common cause of adolescent menorrhagia.[5,6] Thrombocytopenia (platelet count <150 000/μl) has been reported in 13% of 71 girls aged 10–19 years with menorrhagia,[5] including three with newly diagnosed ITP.

Acquired von Willebrand syndrome is a rare condition that occurs in association with autoimmune disorders, endocrine disorders, malignancies and lympho- and myeloproliferative disorders. Acquired von Willebrand syndrome associated with hypothyroidism has been described as predominantly affecting women.[7] The bleeding symptoms, including menorrhagia, are usually mild and respond to thyroid treatment.

Menorrhagia

Heavy menstruation has been reported in women known to have bleeding disorders but it has always been presumed that bleeding disorders are a rare cause of menorrhagia, especially in adults. Since 1998 there has been increasing research interest as well as increasing clinical awareness in this area. The prevalence of bleeding disorders in older women with menorrhagia seems to be underestimated. Identifying bleeding problems in women with menorrhagia and close collaboration between gynaecologists and haematologists in their management is the way forward to improve quality of life and avoid unnecessary surgical interventions.

BLEEDING DISORDERS AS AN UNDERLYING CAUSE OF MENORRHAGIA

Bleeding disorders, particularly von Willebrand's disorder, have been found to be the underlying cause of menorrhagia in a small but significant proportion of women. The prevalence of von Willebrand's disorder in women with menorrhagia was 13% in one systematic review that included 11 studies and 988 women of reproductive age (Table 6.1).[8] The prevalence in individual studies ranged from 5% to 24%, with higher prevalence in European studies (18%; 95% CI 14.5–22.7%) compared with north American studies (10%; 95% CI 7.5–12.9%; $P = 0.007$). This difference was explained by the differences in the ethnic mix of the study populations, criteria used to diagnose menorrhagia and von Willebrand's disorder in individual studies. Underlying bleeding disorders, mainly platelet dysfunction and von Willebrand's disorder, were found in 47% of 115 women with menorrhagia.[40] Adolescents and perimenopausal-age women with menorrhagia were just as likely to have bleeding disorders as were women aged 20–44 years. The results of these studies indicate that bleeding disorders are frequently found in women with menorrhagia and suggest appropriate haemostatic evaluation, regardless of age.

DIAGNOSIS AND ASSESSMENT

Diagnosis of inherited bleeding disorders in women with menorrhagia has several medical implications. First, it enhances rapid and effective medical treatment of menorrhagia. Second, if any surgical intervention becomes necessary, the risk of bleeding complications can be prevented by appropriate preoperative assessment and prophylactic treatment when indicated. Lastly, it has genetic implications and helps the management of any future pregnancies.

There is no consensus among gynaecologists whether testing either for inherited bleeding disorder or only for Von Willebrand's disorder, the most common disorder, should be part of routine investigation in menorrhagia. The RCOG guidelines[9] for the management of menorrhagia recommend testing only when features present in the history or examination are suggestive of bleeding disorders (Grade C recommendation). The American College of Obstetricians and Gynecologists guidelines[10] recommend screening for Von Willebrand's disorder in all adolescents with menorrhagia, but all adults with no pelvic pathology, and all women prior to hysterectomy. Although pelvic pathology, especially fibroids, is common in women of reproductive age, the prevalence of Von Willebrand's disorder in women with pelvic pathology is unknown.

Other less common clotting factor deficiencies such as FVII, FX and FXI deficiency and platelet function defects, as well as fibrinolytic disorders, can be the underlying cause of menorrhagia. Therefore, testing for these disorders is worth considering in high risk groups (e.g. FXI in Jewish women) and in unexplained menorrhagia with normal VWF levels, especially in those with other bleeding symptoms or prolonged bleeding time.

Taking a comprehensive bleeding history may be helpful in identifying women who are likely to have a bleeding disorder. There should be a high index of suspicion of a bleeding disorder in women with:

Table 6.1 Prevalence studies of Von Willebrand's disorder in women presenting with menorrhagia to gynaecologists

Study	Ref.	Women (n)	VWD (n)	Prevalence (%)	95% CI	Age (y) median	Race (%) White	Black	Other	Blood group (%) O	Non-O
Europe											
Edlund et al.	32	30	6	20	7.7–38.5	39	100	–	–	NA	NA
Kadir et al.	33	150	20	13.3	8.3–19.8	39	59	15	12	41	59
Woo et al.	34	38	5	13.1	4.4–28.5	49.0*	100	–	–	NA	NA
Krause et al.	35	153	37	24.2	17.6–31.8	36	NA	NA	NA	NA	NA
Total Europe		**371**	**68**	**18.2**	**14.5–22.7**						
North America											
Kouides et al.	21	178	31	17.4	12.1–23.8	40	80	15	5	53	47
Hambleton et al.	36	118	6	5.1	1.9–10.7	35	65	14	12	48	52
Goodman-Gruen & Hollenbach	37	19	1	5.3	0.1–1.26	39.6*	68	–	32	NA	NA
Dilley et al.	38	121	8	6.6	2.9–12.6	35.5*	36	57	7	49	51
Philip et al.	39,40	74	5	6.7	2.2–15.1	40.0*	70	22	8	59	41
Total North America		**510**	**51**	**10**	**7.5–12.9**						
Other											
Baindur et al.	41	32	5	15.6	5.3–32.8	24.0*	–	–	100	NA	NA
El Ekiaby et al.	42	75	7	9.3	3.8–18.3	NA	–	–	100	NA	NA
Overall total		**988**	**131**	**13.2**	**11.2–115.5**						

* mean; NA = not available; VWD = von Willebrand's disorder

- long-standing menorrhagia
- menorrhagia since menarche
- history of postpartum haemorrhage
- history of postoperative bleeding
- history of bleeding after tooth extraction.

However, the clinical severity of bleeding disorders may vary considerably and menorrhagia may be the only clinical manifestation.

Diagnosis of inherited bleeding disorders is difficult. Genetic diagnosis is the definitive method but is only possible in a small number of cases such as carriers of haemophilia with known family mutation. The diagnosis in the majority of disorders is made on a clinical basis and on laboratory results of coagulation screen and clotting factor (VWF:Ag, VWF:Ac, FVIII:C) assays. However, clinical expression of the disease is variable and the factor levels may overlap with the normal range, especially of mild forms, making the diagnosis difficult and complex. Bleeding time and APTT are prolonged only in people with severe deficiencies. In people with mild VWD, factor levels may be normal, but on repeated testing at least one abnormal value is usually observed. VWF:Ac assay is the single most sensitive assay for screening for most forms of VWD. Because of the variability of laboratory findings in VWD, repeated testing to establish the diagnosis of mild VWD is

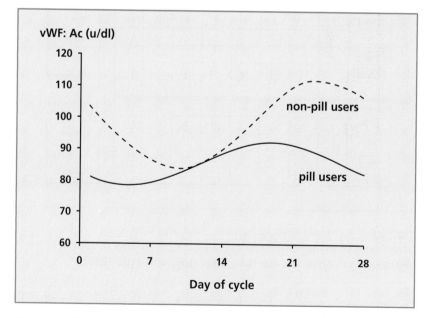

Figure 6.1 Variation of VWF activity levels over a 28-day cycle in oral contraceptive pill users and nonusers

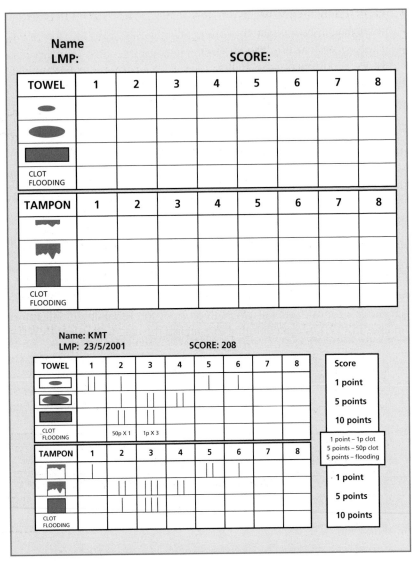

Figure 6.2 Pictorial blood assessment chart and scoring system for assessment of menstrual blood loss; an example of how to complete the chart, using the detailed scoring system (Higham *et al.*, 1990).[14]

recommended especially with borderline levels. Restricting sampling to early follicular phase is recommended as factor levels fluctuate during the menstrual cycle (Figure 6.1).[11]

MENORRHAGIA IN WOMEN WITH BLEEDING DISORDERS

The high prevalence of menorrhagia among women with Von Willebrand's disorder has been reported in several studies. In a survey of 99 women with type 1 Von Willebrand's disorder from four haemophilia centres in the USA, 78% reported heavy periods, 71% required medical attention and 15% required hysterectomy.[12] In a study by Ragni *et al.*,[13] 93% of the 38 women with Von Willebrand's disorder suffered from heavy menstruation. Menorrhagia was also the most common initial bleeding symptom leading to the diagnosis of the disease in 53%, and in all the women this had started at menarche.

Women with bleeding disorders may consider heavy menstruation as normal and may not seek medical advice because menorrhagia usually starts from menarche. In addition, because of the hereditary nature of bleeding disorders, mothers and sisters in the family may also have excessive menstrual blood loss. Therefore, these women should regularly be asked about their periods and menstrual loss should be assessed. The pictorial blood assessment chart (PBAC)[14] (Figure 6.2), a simple non-laboratory method for semi-quantitative measure of menstrual blood loss, is helpful for initial assessment and monitoring response to treatment.

Menstrual loss was assessed using a PBAC in women with inherited bleeding disorders (VWD, mainly type 1; FXI deficiency; and carriers of haemophilia). The incidence of menorrhagia, defined by a PBAC score of more than 100, was 73%, 57% and 59% respectively, compared with 29% in the age matched control group. These women also had prolonged menstruation and 25% of them bled for more than 8 days compared with

Table 6.2 Menstrual scores in women with inherited bleeding disorders and in the control group

	Median score	Range	Women with score >100
Carriers of haemophilia A (n = 14)	111	50–482	8 (57.1%)
Carriers of Haemophilia B (n = 7)	115	53–200	4 (57.1%)
VWD (n = 57)	139	55–456	42 (73.7%)
FXI deficiency (n = 17)	108	38–424	10 (58.8%)
Total (n = 95)	122	38–482	64 (67.4%)*
Control (n = 69)	73	9–310	20 (29.0%)*

n = number of women completed PBAC; * = statistically significant difference (p = 0.001) only 4% in the control group.[15] Table 6.2 demonstrates menstrual scores in the different groups. In the same study, a strong relationship between menstrual blood loss and duration of menstruation was also demonstrated (Figure 6.3), which indicates that these women bleed heavily throughout menstruation. This is in contrast to women with menorrhagia without bleeding disorders, where it has been shown that 90% of the total menses is lost in the first 3 days.[16]

Although menorrhagia in women with inherited bleeding disorders is likely to be due to the clotting factor deficiency, each individual should have appropriate gynaecological assessment to exclude local causes, especially the possibility of malignancy in older women.

Menorrhagia is also a major cause of iron deficiency anaemia. This type of anaemia was reported in 64% of 81 menstruating women with type 1 Von Willebrand's disorder compared with 34% in a menstruating control group.[12] The hysterectomy rate among these women is also high and was 14% among 431 women studied by four groups of investigators.[12,13,15,17]

Hysterectomy is usually done at a young age. The mean age of hysterectomy at the Royal Free Hospital was 38 years and in the majority hysterectomy was performed before the diagnosis of Von Willebrand's disorder. In types 2 and 3, the risk is even higher and the rate of hysterectomy was reported to be 23%.[18]

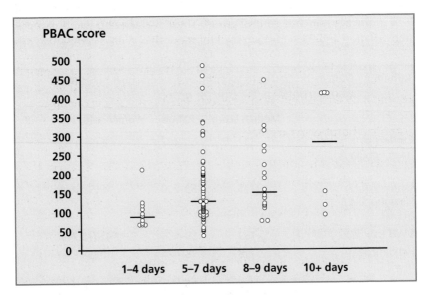

Figure 6.3 Relationship between menstrual scores and duration of menstruation. Horizontal lines represent median values

Management of gynaecological problems in women with bleeding disorders

This requires close collaboration between gynaecologists and a haemophilia centre. Ideally, these women should be managed in a combined clinic, where expertise and facilities are available to provide comprehensive assessment of their bleeding disorders and gynaecological problems as well as a management plan.

TREATMENT OF MENORRHAGIA IN WOMEN WITH INHERITED BLEEDING DISORDERS

Medical treatment

The treatment of menorrhagia is usually medical. The most commonly used first-line options are tranexamic acid, combined oral contraceptive compounds or DDAVP by intranasal spray or self-administered subcutaneous injection. The choice is dependent upon the woman's age, reproductive state, preference and availability of the medications, as well as the clinician's experience and preference.

Tranexamic acid

Tranexamic acid is an antifibrinolytic agent that reduces endometrial tissue plasminogen activator activity and antigen and thus reduces menstrual blood loss in women with menorrhagia. A 54% reduction in menstrual blood loss was reported in a randomised controlled study.[19] The adverse effects of tranexamic acid are minimal and include nausea, headache and dizziness. There has been some concern about its thrombotic complications, although a 2001 study showed no increased risk of thrombosis in women.[20] Tranexamic acid is effective, safe and far less expensive than other treatment modalities and should be considered as a first line therapy.

Combined oral contraceptives

Combined oral contraceptives control the menstrual cycle and inhibit endometrial growth as well as increasing FVIII:C and VWF:Ac levels. They are commonly used for women, especially adolescents, with inherited bleeding disorders and menorrhagia. However, their efficacy in reducing the menstrual loss in women with bleeding disorders is unknown; no increase in FVIII and VWF was seen with low dose (30 μg oestradiol) pills.[11] In women with type 1 VWD, a standard dose of oral contraceptive was subjectively effective only 24% of the time while high-dose oral contraceptive therapy was effective only 37% of the time.[12] In types 2 and 3 VWD, 88% of women with menorrhagia stated that combined oral contraceptives were effective.[18] Oral contraceptives have the added benefit of regular menstrual cycles and excellent contraception. On the other hand, they are associated with the risk of thrombosis. Women with bleeding disorders, however, have low thrombotic risk.

DDAVP (desmopressin) nasal spray

DDAVP (1-desamino-8-D-arginine vasopressin) is a vasopressin analogue. It causes a rapid release of FVIII and VWF from endothelial cells thus increasing their plasma concentration. It is particularly effective in patients with type 1 Von Willebrand's disorder and mild to moderate haemophilia A. Women with type 2A Von Willebrand's disorder may also respond to DDAVP. In type 2B Von Willebrand's disorder, a rare subtype, DDAVP may induce thrombocytopenia and is therefore considered contra-indicated for the management of these women. Women with type 3 Von Willebrand's disorder do not respond to DDAVP. DDAVP is an important therapeutic alternative to plasma-derived coagulation products because it avoids the risk of infection with blood-borne viruses. A test dose must be performed prior to treatment to differentiate responders from non-responders. Adverse effects of DDAVP are few, usually mild tachycardia, headache and flushing due to its vasomotor effects. There is also a slight risk of hyponatraemia and water intoxication as DDAVP has an anti-diuretic effect. This complication can be greatly reduced by strict fluid

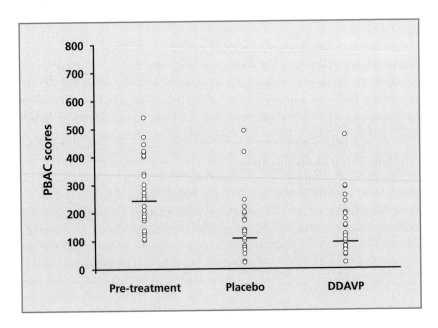

Figure 6.4 Menstrual scores: pretreatment, placebo and DDAVP treated periods; horizontal lines represent median values

restriction and electrolyte monitoring, especially in those receiving several doses of DDAVP.

Home treatment with DDAVP is now available and is used for menorrhagia. DDAVP is administered as a nasal spray or by subcutaneous injection. The response of DDAVP nasal spray was considered by 68 women with Von Willebrand's disorder and menorrhagia to be good or excellent during 92% of the time of use.[21] The mean duration of menstrual bleeding was decreased in women with Von Willebrand's disorder, carriers of haemophilia A or platelet disorders.[22] In the only randomised study using PBAC for assessment of menstrual blood loss, there was a significant decrease in PBAC scores with DDAVP compared with pretreatment, although the difference was not statistically significant compared with placebo treatment (Figure 6.4).[23] Based on the findings that 90% of all menstrual flow is in the first 3 days,[16] DDAVP nasal spray is usually given in the first 2–3 days of the period. However, as women with bleeding disorders bleed heavily throughout their menstruation[11] the dose and duration should be tailored according to the woman's PBAC.

Other medical treatments

Progestogens are widely used in the treatment of dysfunctional uterine bleeding despite the limited evidence to support this. This treatment modality may be useful in high doses, orally or in the form of a parenteral progestogen-only contraceptive, alone or in combination with DDAVP or factor concentrate, to arrest acute haemorrhage. Cyclical progesterones are only effective in the management of menorrhagia if used from days 5–26 of the cycle and considered as a second line of treatment for women with inherited bleeding disorders not responding to the above treatments or when these treatments are contraindicated. Compliance with this regimen is usually poor.

Other medical treatments including danazol and gonadotrophin-releasing hormone agonists are used with reasonable efficacy in the treatment of menorrhagia in general. However, experience regarding their effectiveness in women with inherited bleeding disorders is lacking in the literature. In addition, the adverse effects and risks associated with a long-term hypo-oestrogenic state make them unacceptable for long-term usage. Gonadotrophin-releasing hormone agonists with add-back therapy with tibolone 2.5 mg may be an alternative to surgery for women with severe bleeding disorders such as type 3 Von Willebrand's disorder not responding to other treatments.

Levonorgestrel intrauterine system

The levonorgestrel intrauterine system (LNG-IUS), is highly effective in reducing menstrual loss. However, there is a lack of published data on the use and effectiveness of this system in menorrhagia due to bleeding disorders. Owing to the high local level of progestogens, the use of this hormone-releasing system is associated with suppression of endometrial growth and spiral arterioles as well as capillary thrombosis. In addition, it has no effect on endometrial factor VIII activity, which is reduced by ordinary intrauterine contraceptive devices.[24] In one study,[25] the Mirena® intrauterine system was assessed in 16 women with bleeding disorders and menorrhagia not responding to medical treatment. After insertion, all women had irregular spotting ranging from 30 to 90 days. Eleven women did not think that the irregular bleeding affected their lives, while the remaining five were only slightly affected. At nine-month follow-up, nine women had become amenorrhoeic. In the remaining six, the menstrual loss was significantly reduced from a median PBAC score of 213 to one of 47 ($P = 0.0001$). Quality of life during menstruation was improved and none reported any adverse effects.

The main problem with LNG-IUS is a high discontinuation rate (20% in randomised controlled trials, and 17% in case series reviewed by Stewart *et al.*[26] because of irregular bleeding during the first 3–6 months and the progestogenic adverse effects. Proper counselling and patient education may increase tolerance. The LNG-IUS is an effective and a reversible method of contraception, which is an added advantage, especially in women who wish to preserve their fertility. In women with bleeding disorders, this method should be considered prior to any surgical management.

SURGICAL MANAGEMENT

Surgical intervention is sometimes required in women unresponsive to medical treatment. Surgical procedures, even relatively minor operations such as hysteroscopy and diagnostic curettage, can be complicated by haemorrhage in women with inherited bleeding disorders. Therefore, good liaison between the local haemophilia centre and the surgical and anaesthetic team is essential. Factor levels should be checked pre-operatively and adequate haemostatic cover provided with the aim of maintaining the clotting factors greater than 50 iu/dl for major surgery and greater than 30 iu/dl for minor surgery until healing is complete. Treatment may need to continue postoperatively, sometimes for up to 10 days, to reduce the development of secondary haematomas. Any surgical intervention should be carried out by a senior gynaecologist; a technique with least risk of bleeding should be chosen; bleeding vessels should be ligated and not cauterised as oozing can occur after surgery; and the use of surgical drains should be considered. It is also important to remember that excessive bleeding may be surgical rather than a result of a failure of adequate replacement therapy. Monitoring postoperatively is continued depending upon the nature of the operation and the factor level of the patient. Secondary haemorrhage is not uncommon and, for major surgery, treatment and inpatient observation may be necessary for 7–10 days. Unexplained operative and postoperative bleeding that does not respond to general measures should always alert the gynaecologist to the possibility of an underlying bleeding disorder as a causative factor.

Hysterectomy is the definitive treatment and has the highest patient satisfaction. However, it is a major operation and associated with a mortality of 0.3 per 1000 and 3% serious morbidity.[27] Endometrial ablative techniques are increasingly used for management of menorrhagia not responding to medical treatment. Endometrial ablation is associated with shorter operative time, fewer complications and faster return to normal activity and work. Thermal or laser ablation may be preferred in women with bleeding disorders because of the risk of haemorrhage with endometrial resection. More recently, non-hysteroscopic techniques (microwave ablation, thermal balloon ablation, hydrothermal ablation, cryoablation and others) have become available. These techniques are simpler to learn and are quicker and safer procedures. The need for fluid distension media, and its associated risks, is avoided. In addition, they can be performed under local anaesthesia as an outpatient procedure. Toth *et al.*[28] evaluated the effectiveness of a thermal uterine balloon therapy system in a group of women with multiple morbidity. Twenty-five of 70 women had coagulopathy. No serious complications occurred during or after the procedure and the success rate 36 months after the procedure was over 90%. This simple procedure appears to have reproducible results whatever the surgeon's skill. Clearly, the second-generation techniques for dysfunctional uterine bleeding can be proposed under local anaesthesia to minimise the risks and the success rate is always over 80–90%. Thus, hysterectomy must become the last option, with very few indications.

DYSMENORRHOEA AND MID-CYCLE PAIN

Moderate to severe dysmenorrhoea has been reported in approximately half of 180 women from the Royal Free Hospital and from the north of New York State.[12,29] Nonsteroidal anti-inflammatory drugs are used successfully for dysmenorrhoea and may also reduce menstrual blood loss in women with menorrhagia. In women with bleeding disorders, especially those with severe deficiency, they may increase menstrual blood loss and cause other bleeding complications because of their anti-platelet effect. Their use in these women, therefore, is inappropriate.

Mid-cycle pain (Mittelschmerz syndrome), as severe as their menstrual pain, was reported in 49% of 81 women with type 1 Von Willebrand's disorder studied by Kouides *et al.*[12] This pain probably arises from ovulation with subsequent haemorrhage into the corpus luteum or peritoneal irritation due to bleeding from the edges of a recently formed corpus luteum. Acute abdomen due to haemoperitoneum as well as extension of bleeding into the broad ligament with spontaneous rupture of corpus luteum has been reported in women with bleeding disorders.[30,31] Although a rare complication, it is an important one to consider in these women, especially those with severe deficiency such as type 3 Von Willebrand's disorder, before embarking on any surgical intervention, as conservative management with factor replacement is usually effective and obviates the need for surgery.

Quality of life

Menorrhagia and dysmenorrhoea adversely affect women's quality of life and may have a major influence on lifestyle and employment. In a study at the Royal Free Hospital, women with inherited bleeding disorders had a significantly worse quality of life during menstruation compared with the control group. Quality of life was worst among women with Von Willebrand's disorder, especially those who passed clots, suffered flooding and had prolonged menstruation. Between 39% and 46% of these women lost time from work.[11,12] They also accomplished less and experienced difficulties performing their work. A strong relationship was found between gynaecological history and psychological problems among 181 women with Von Willebrand's disorder;[17] 28% of the women in the same study met the criteria for anxiety disorders.

Key points

- Undiagnosed bleeding disorders, especially Von Willebrand's disorder, can be the under-lying cause of menorrhagia in a significant proportion of women.
- Testing for Von Willebrand's disorder should be part of investigations for women with menorrhagia before embarking on any surgical intervention for diagnosis or treatment.
- A detailed bleeding history is crucial to identify those women who require detailed haematological investigations.
- Close collaboration with haematologists is required in the management of women with menorrhagia, when a bleeding disorder is suspected or diagnosed.
- Women with bleeding disorders suffer significant gynaecological morbidity, including menorrhagia, dysmenorrhea and mid-cycle pain that can affect their health and quality of life.
- Increased awareness among clinicians of these problems and the treatment options available is essential to improve quality of life and avoid unnecessary surgical intervention.
- Tranexamic acid is a safe, effective and inexpensive treatment for menorrhagia in these women and should be considered as first-line management.
- DDAVP nasal spray increases VWF and FVIII and can be used as a home treatment for some women with bleeding disorders. A test dose is required to assess response.
- Levonorgestrel intrauterine system should be considered prior to surgery.
- When contemplating gynaecological surgery in these women, a multi-disciplinary team approach is required to minimise bleeding complications.

References

1   Rizza CR, Rhymes IL, Austen DE, Kernoff PB, Aroni SA. Detection of carriers of haemophilia: a 'blind' study. *Br J Haematol* 1975;30(4):447–56.

2   Lyon MF. Sex chromatin and gene action in the mammalian X-chromosome. *Am J Hum Genet* 1962;14:135–48.

3   Seligsohn U. Factor XI deficiency. *Thromb Haemost* 1993;70(1):68–71.

4   Bolton-Maggs PH, Young Wan-Yin B, McCraw A, Slack J, Kernoff, P. Inheritance and bleeding in factor XI-deficiency. *Br J Haematol* 1988;69:521–8.

5   Bevan JA, Maloney KW, Gill JC, Montgomery RR, Scott JP. Bleeding causes of menorrhagia in adolescents. *J Pediatr* 2001;138:856–61.

6   Claessens EA, Cowell CA. Acute adolescent menorrhagia. *Am J Obstet Gynecol* 1981;139(3):277–80.

7 Nitu-Whaley IC, Lee CA. Acquired von Willebrand syndrome: report of 10 cases and review of literature. *Haemophilia* 1999;5:318–29.

8 Shakar M, Lee CA, Sabin CA, Economides DL, Kadir RA. Von Willibrand disease in women with menorrhagia: a systematic review. *BJOG* 2004;111:734–40.

9 Royal College of Obstetricians and Gynaecologists. *The Initial Management of Menorrhagia*. Evidence-Based Clinical Guidelines No. 1. London: RCOG; 1998.

10 American College of Obstetricians and Gynecologists. *Von Willebrand's Disease in Gynecologic Practice*. Committee Opinion No 263. Washington DC: ACOG; 2001.

11 Kadir RA, Economides DL, Sabin CA, Owens D, Lee CA. Variations in coagulation factors in women: Effect of age, ethnicity, menstrual cycle and combined oral contraceptive. *Thromb Haemost* 1999;82:1456–61.

12 Kouides P, Phatak P, Burkhart P, *et al.* Gynaecological and obstetrical morbidity in women with Type 1 von Willebrand disease: Results of a patient survey. *Haemophilia* 2000;6:643–8.

13 Ragni MV, Bontempo FA, Cortese Hasset A. Von Willebrand disease and bleeding in women. *Haemophilia* 1999;5:313–17.

14 Higham JM, O'Brien PM, Shaw RW. Assessment of menstrual blood loss using a pictorial chart. *Br J Obstet Gynaecol* 1990;97(8):734–9.

15 Kadir RA, Economides DL, Sabin CA, Pollard D, Lee CA. Assessment of menstrual blood loss and gynaecological problems in patients with inherited bleeding disorders. *Haemophilia* 1999;5:40–48.

16 Janssen CA, Scholten PC, Heintz AP. A simple visual assessment technique to discriminate between menorrhagia and normal menstrual blood loss. *Obstet Gynecol* 1995;85(6):977–82.

17 Rozeik CH, Scharrer I. Gynecological disorders and psychological problems in 184 women with von Willebrand disease. *Haemophilia* 1998;4:293.

18 Foster PA. The reproductive health of women with von Willebrand Disease unresponsive to DDAVP: results of an international survey. On behalf of the Subcommittee on von Willebrand Factor of the Scientific and Standardization Committee of the ISTH. *Thromb Haemost* 1995;74(2):784–90.

19 Bonnar J, Sheppard BL. Treatment of menorrhagia during menstruation: randomised controlled trial of ethamsylate, mefenamic acid, and tranexamic acid. *Br Med J* 1996;313(7057):579–82.

20 Berntorp E, Follrud C, Lethagen S. No increased risk of venous thrombosis in women taking tranexamic acid. *Thromb Haemost* 2001;86:714–15.

21 Kouides P, Burkhart P, Phatak P, *et al.* Type 1 von Willebrand disease causes significant obstetric–gynaecological morbidity. *Blood* 1997;90 Suppl 1:32a.

22 Lethagen S, Ragnarson TG. Self-treatment with desmopressin intranasal spray in patients with bleeding disorders: effect on bleeding symptoms and socioeconomic factors. *Ann Hematol* 1993;66(5):257–60.

23 Kadir RA, Lee CA, Pollard D, Economides DL. DDAVP nasal spray for treatment of menorrhagia in women with inherited bleeding disorders: A randomised placebo controlled cross-over study. *Haemophilia* 2002;8:787–93.

24 Zhu P, Hongzhi L, Wenliang S. Observation of the activity of factor VIII in the endometrium of women pre- and post-insertion of three types of IUDs. *Contraception* 1991;44:367–87.

25 Kingman CE, Kadir RA, Lee CA, Economides DL. The use of levonorgestrel-releasing intrauterine system for the treatment of menorrhagia in women with inherited bleeding disorders. *BJOG* 2004;111:1425–8.

26 Stewart A, Cummins C, Gold L, Jordan R, Phillips W. The effectiveness of the levonorgestrel-releasing intrauterine system in menorrhagia: a systematic review. *BJOG* 2001;108:74–86.

27 Maresh M, Metcalfe M, McPherson K. The VALUE national hysterectomy study: description of patients and their surgery. *BJOG* 2002;109:302–12.

28 Toth D, Gervaise A, Guzel D, Fernandez H. Thermal balloon ablation in patients with multiple morbidity: 3 years follow-up. *J Am Soc Gynecol Laparosc* 2004;11:236–9.

29 Kadir, R. A., Sabin, C. A., Pollard, D., Lee, C. A., Economides, D. L. Quality of life during menstruation in patients with inherited bleeding disorders. *Haemophilia* 1998;4:836–841.

30 Greer IA, Lowe GD, Walker JJ, Forbes CD. Haemorrhagic problems in obstetrics and gynaecology in patients with congenital coagulopathies. *Br J Obstet Gynaecol* 1991;98(9):909–18.

31 Gomez A, Lucia JF, Perella M, Aguilar C. Haemoperitoneum caused by haemorrhagic corpus luteum in a patient with type 3 von Willebrand's disease. *Haemophilia* 1998;4(1):60–62.

32 Edlund M, Blomback M, von Schoultz B, Andersson O. On the value of menorrhagia as a predictor for coagulation disorders. *Am J Hematol* 1996;53(4):234–8.

33 Kadir, R. A., Economides, D. L., Sabin, C. A., Owens, D., Lee, C. A. Frequency of inherited bleeding disorders in women with menorrhagia. *Lancet* 1998;351:485–489.

34 Woo Y, White B, Corbally R, *et al.* von Willebrand disease: an important cause of dysfunctional uterine bleeding. *Blood Coagul Fibrinol* 2002;13:89–93.

35 Krause M, Aygoren-Pursun E, Ehrenforth S, Ludwig G, Vigh TH, Scharrer I. Coagulation disorders in women with menorrhagia. *Haemophilia* 2000;6:245.

36 Hambleton J, Roth J, Jumack-Dewell J, Schwartz B, Seremetis S. Prevalence of von Willebrand disease in women with menorrhagia: a preliminary report. *Haemophilia* 2000;6:242.

37 Goodman-Gruen D, Hollenbach K. The prevalence of von Willebrand disease in women with abnormal uterine bleeding. *J Womens Health Gend Based Med* 2001;10:677–80.

38 Dilley A, Drews C, Miller C, *et al.* von Willebrand disease and other inherited bleeding disorders in women with diagnosed menorrhagia. *Obstet Gynecol* 2001;97:630–36.

39 Philipp C, Faiz A, Dowling N, *et al.* Age and the prevalence of bleeding disorders in women with menorrhagia. *Obstet Gynecol* 2005;105:61–6.

40 Baindur S, Shetty S, Pathare AV, *et al.* Screening for von Willebrand's disease in patients with menorrhagia. *Haemophilia* 2000;6:240–1.

41 El Ekiaby M, Ahmed A, Farang O, Khattab D. Von Willebrand's disease as a cause of menorrhagia. *Haemophilia* 2002;8:512–14.

7 Venous thromboembolism in obstetrics and gynaecology

Venous thromboembolism (VTE) describes thrombotic events that occur in the venous circulation, encompassing primary thrombosis and embolic events such as pulmonary embolism (PTE).

VTE is a common cause of morbidity and mortality. Thromboses most commonly occur in the deep veins of the lower limbs (DVT), but can arise at other sites such as the upper limbs or mesenteric vessels. DVT may go unrecognised before presentation with PTE. In people hospitalised after trauma, surgery or immobilising medical illness, the risk of VTE is increased ten-fold,[1] and PTE is a significant cause of death. Pulmonary embolism remains the leading cause of direct maternal death in the UK.[2]

Following a treated DVT, over 60% of women have objectively confirmed deep venous insufficiency, and almost 80% will develop post-thrombotic syndrome. The odds ratio for developing venous insufficiency after a DVT has been estimated at 10.9 (95% CI 4.2–28.0) compared with 3.8 (95% CI 1.2–12.3) after a PTE.[3] The difference may be due to thrombus clearing from the legs in PTE, leading to less extensive damage to the deep venous system. Other long-term effects of DVT include a significant risk of recurrent thrombosis, restriction of contraceptive choice and complications of anticoagulant therapy, while PTE carries a risk of subsequent pulmonary hypertension.

Epidemiology

VTE occurs in approximately 0.1% of pregnancies, with a two-fold increase in risk for those over the age of 35 years.[4] The CEMD indicates that the incidence of fatal PTE has fallen substantially from the early 1950s. The greatest reduction has occurred in deaths following vaginal delivery. The number of antenatal and intrapartum deaths also remains relatively static despite major advances in identification of risk, thromboprophylaxis, diagnosis and treatment. Deaths following caesarean section changed little from the 1950s until publication of the Royal College of Obstetricians and Gynaecologists guideline on thromboprophylaxis[5] in 1995 after which the number of deaths fell dramatically, although they have risen again in last triennium.[2] This highlights the effectiveness of appropriate thromboprophylaxis following caesarean section and perhaps more importantly emphasises the need for better prophylaxis in the antenatal period and after vaginal delivery.

The incidence of DVT following gynaecological surgery appears comparable to that associated with general abdominal surgery. Estimates of incidence range from 4–38% (average 16%) in unprotected patients, with fatal PTE reported in around 0.4%.[6]

Pathophysiology

Virchow's classic triad of factors underlying venous thrombosis, namely hypercoagulability, venous stasis and vascular damage, all occur in normal pregnancy and delivery (see Chapter 1), and in gynaecological surgery. In pregnancy, venous flow, as measured by ultrasound, falls substantially by the end of the first trimester, progressing to around a 50% reduction by the end

Table 7.1 Risk factors for venous thromboembolism in hospital patients

Patient factors	Disease or surgical procedure
Age	Trauma or surgery to the pelvis or lower limb
Obesity	Malignancy, particularly pelvic or intra-abdominal or metastatic
Varicose veins	Cardiac failure
Deep venous insufficiency	Recent myocardial infarction
Immobility	Paralysis of lower limbs
Pregnancy	Infection
Puerperium	Inflammatory bowel disease
Hormone therapy	Nephrotic syndrome
Previous VTE	Polycythaemia
Thrombophilia:	Paroxysmal nocturnal haemoglobinuria
Antithrombin Deficiency	Behcet's disease
Protein C deficiency	Paraproteinaemia
Protein S deficiency	
Factor V Leiden	
Prothrombin gene variant	
Homocystinaemia	
Lupus anticoagulant	
Antiphospholipid antibodies	

modified from SIGN[1]

of the second trimester, reaching a nadir at 36 weeks and taking around 6 weeks to return to nonpregnant flow rates.[7] Endothelial damage to pelvic vessels can occur during vaginal delivery, caesarean section or gynaecological surgery. Specific coexistent disease or surgical factors may provide additional risk (Table 7.1). Multiple risk factors may be present in many women. Age over 35 years, body mass index (BMI) greater than 30 kg/m^2, previous VTE and thrombophilia are particularly important risk factors. In women with previous VTE, screening for inherited and acquired thrombophilia should be considered. Thrombophilia is discussed in Chapter 8.

In pregnancy, more than 70% of DVT are located in the ileofemoral region, compared with only 9% in nonpregnant women. This is important, as ileofemoral DVT are more likely to generate PTE than isolated calf vein thrombosis. Almost 90% of DVT affect the left side in pregnancy compared with 55% in nonpregnant women.[8] This may be due to compression of the left iliac vein by the right iliac and ovarian arteries, which cross the vein on the left side only.

Methods of antithrombotic prophylaxis and treatment

Many therapeutic agents may be used in the management of VTE. The choice of agent and dosage is determined by the setting (prophylaxis or treatment of an acute event), balance of risks and benefit, and individual patient factors such as allergy or co-morbidity.

HEPARIN

Unfractionated heparin (UFH) or low-molecular-weight heparin (LMWH) are the anticoagulants of choice in pregnancy due to the fetal hazards of coumarins. In contrast to warfarin, neither UFH[9] nor LMWH cross the placenta[10,11] and there is no evidence of teratogenesis or risk of fetal haemorrhage.[12]

Prolonged use of UFH can be associated with symptomatic osteoporosis (with around a 2% incidence of osteoporotic fractures), allergy and heparin-induced thrombocytopenia.[13] LMWHs may have a lower risk of osteoporosis.[14]

Heparin-induced thrombocytopenia is rare but life threatening. It is an idiosyncratic immune mediated reaction associated with extensive venous thrombosis that usually occurs between 5 and 15 days after the institution of heparin. The risk has been estimated at 1–3% with UFH and is substantially lower with LMWH.[15] Allergic reactions usually take the form of itchy, erythematous lesions at injection sites and should be distinguished from faulty injection technique with associated bruising. Switching heparin preparations may be helpful although cross-reactivity can occur. LMWH is the heparin of choice for thromboprophylaxis in pregnancy because of a better adverse effect profile, good safety record for mother and fetus and once daily dosing.[16]

WARFARIN

Warfarin crosses the placenta and is a teratogen. Warfarin embryopathy (midface hypoplasia, stippled chondral calcification, scoliosis, short proximal limbs and short phalanges) can occur in around 4–5% of cases exposed between 6 and 9 weeks of gestation.[17] The risk is increased when the dose of warfarin is greater than 5 mg/day.[18] As the fetal liver is immature and levels of vitamin K-dependent coagulation factors low, maternal warfarin therapy maintained in the therapeutic range will be associated with excessive anticoagulation and potential bleeding problems in the fetus. Warfarin should be avoided beyond 36 weeks of gestation[19] because of the excessive bleeding risk to both mother and fetus in the peripartum period.

Warfarin is effective in preventing DVT after major gynaecological surgery. It can be given in a fixed mini-dose regimen,[20] which avoids the haemorrhagic hazards of full anticoagulation. The latter is usually reserved for high risk patients because of the increased risk of bleeding and need for daily laboratory monitoring. Spinal and epidural anaesthesia are contraindicated in the presence of full anticoagulation.

DEXTRAN 70

Dextran has significant thromboprophylactic effects. It has been shown to be as effective as LMWH in preventing fatal PTE,[21] and can be administered during and immediately after operation as part of the intravenous fluid regimen. Care must be taken to avoid fluid overload and dextrans should be avoided in patients with renal or cardiac insufficiency. There is a significant risk of allergic reactions including anaphylactic and anaphylactoid reactions.

Dextran should be avoided in pregnancy because of the risk of maternal anaphylactoid reactions, which have been associated with uterine hypertonus, profound fetal distress, and a high incidence of fetal death or profound neurological damage.[22]

ASPIRIN

While it is clear that venous thrombosis occurs as a result of activation of the coagulation system resulting in fibrin formation and deposition, the presence of platelet aggregates has been noted in some early venous thrombi. Thus, drugs suppressing platelet function may be of benefit in preventing venous thrombosis. Clinical trials have demonstrated a significant reduction in fatal PTE (0.2% versus 0.6%; NNT 250) and symptomatic VTE to a lesser extent, although at the expense of a significant increase in major bleeding (7.7% versus 6.2%), and no significant reduction in total mortality (3.9% versus 4.0%).[1] Nevertheless, due to its ease of administration, aspirin may have a role in long-term thromboprophylaxis following discharge from hospital. Aspirin 150 mg/day started preoperatively and continued for 35 days is effective prophylaxis in surgical patients.[1] Aspirin may also have a role in women where other thromboprophylactic measures are unsuitable or contraindicated.

The effectiveness of aspirin in preventing DVT in pregnancy remains to be established and is probably less than LMWH.[23] It may be useful in women unable to take heparin or in whom the balance of risk is not considered sufficient to merit heparin. Low dose (60–75 mg daily) aspirin is not associated with adverse pregnancy outcome in the second and third trimesters.[24,25] Aspirin is effective in the management of recurrent pregnancy loss in the setting of antiphospholipid antibodies (see Chapter 8).

HIRUDIN

Hirudin, a direct thrombin inhibitor used in the nonpregnant for treatment of heparin-induced thrombocytopenia, is also used for postoperative prophylaxis. As it crosses the placenta it should not be used in pregnancy. However, it was not detectable in breast milk in one lactating mother.[26]

MECHANICAL METHODS

The main mechanical methods are intermittent pneumatic calf compression and thromboembolic deterrent graduated elastic compression stockings. Intermittent pneumatic calf compression devices attempt to mimic the muscle pump by gentle intermittent compression of the leg veins, while graduated elastic compression stockings exert a pressure gradient maximum at the ankle, decreasing towards the thigh. The aim of the stockings is to reduce venous stasis, although their precise mode of action is unclear. It has been suggested that they do not increase flow velocity but prevent passive venous dilatation, which has been shown to occur during surgery and may provoke endothelial damage.[27]

Both methods have a significant effect in preventing deep venous thrombosis, although it is not clear whether intermittent pneumatic calf compression devices offer any advantages over graduated elastic compression stockings (Table 7.2). Graduated elastic compression stockings are effective prophylaxis in the nonpregnant and, in view of the pregnancy-related changes in the venous system, could be of considerable value in pregnancy. They can also be employed in acute DVT. Intermittent pneumatic calf compression devices are useful in the perioperative situation (including caesarean section) and immediately postpartum,

Table 7.2 Indirect comparisons of thromboprophylactic measures in elective major general surgery based on routine radio labelled fibrinogen leg scanning

Regimen	Incidence of DVT (%)	
	Mean	95% CI
Untreated controls	25	24–27
LMW heparin	6	6–7
Low dose unfractionated heparin	8	7–8
Graduated elastic compression stockings	14	10–20
Intermittent calf compression	3	1–8
Warfarin	10	3–18
Dextran	16	13–18
Aspirin	20	16–25

modified from SIGN[56] and ACCP[30]

particularly in high risk women. They may be combined with other techniques or used in women where heparin is contraindicated.

Thromboprophylaxis

VTE is a significant cause of morbidity and mortality in both obstetric and gynaecological practice. The identification of risk factors for VTE provides an opportunity for prevention. Evidence exists to suggest that a reduction in events can be achieved with effective thromboprophylaxis in targeted individuals. The choice of method for thromboprophylaxis will be dependent on the combination of a critical assessment of the level of risk in any given situation and the individual woman's preferences.

RECOMMENDATIONS FOR THROMBOPROPHYLAXIS IN PREGNANCY

In general, the potential risk of VTE, including any relevant personal and family history, should be assessed in all women early in pregnancy (or prepregnancy in women already known to be at high risk of VTE) and reviewed if new risk factors arise during pregnancy, labour or postpartum (Table 7.3). Immobilisation during pregnancy, labour and the puerperium should be minimised and dehydration avoided. Graduated elastic compression stockings may be worn in all women at risk of VTE, particularly during hospitalisation. Specific advice is available[28] and should be offered to pregnant women planning air travel, which may increase the risk of VTE.

Table 7.3 Common risk factors for VTE in pregnancy

Age over 35 years

Caesarean section particularly as an emergency in labour

Operative vaginal delivery

High body mass index (>30 kg/m2)

Heritable or acquired thrombophilia

Past history of DVT or PTE

Gross varicose veins

Current infection or inflammatory process (e.g. active inflammatory bowel disease, urinary tract infection)

Pre-eclampsia

Immobility

Significant current medical problem (e.g. nephrotic syndrome, cardiac failure)

Paraplegia

Women with two or more current persisting risk factors (Table 7.3) undergoing vaginal delivery and all women undergoing caesarean section, especially emergency caesarean section, are at increased risk of VTE and should receive prophylactic LMWH for 3–5 days following delivery. Any woman with three or more risk factors should receive antenatal thromboprophylaxis with LMWH and postnatal thromboprophylaxis for at least 3–5 days following delivery. Antenatal prophylaxis (subcutaneous LMWH e.g. 40 mg enoxaparin or 5000 iu dalteparin daily) should be started early in pregnancy or as soon as increased risk is identified. Anti-Xa monitoring is generally not necessary. However, adjustments should be made to the dose for women with low (<50 kg) body weight (e.g. 20 mg enoxaparin or 2500 iu dalteparin daily) and importantly for obese women (early pregnancy BMI >30) who may require higher doses of LMWH – these women will require Anti-Xa monitoring and should be managed with the help of a haematologist.

At least 12 hours should elapse between the last prophylactic dose of LMWH heparin and the introduction or removal of an epidural or spinal catheter.

Use of heparin or warfarin does not preclude breastfeeding. Heparins are not secreted in breast milk. Warfarin is not secreted in breast milk in clinically significant amounts and is safe to use during lactation.

THROMBOPROPHYLAXIS IN PREGNANT WOMEN WITH PREVIOUS VTE OR KNOWN THROMBOPHILIA

Single previous VTE

There is clinical consensus that women with more than one previous VTE should receive antenatal thromboprophylaxis, but management of a single previous event is more controversial. There is some evidence that women with a previous VTE associated with a temporary risk factor, not pregnancy related and with no additional risk factor or identifiable thrombophilia, should not routinely receive antenatal thromboprophylaxis.[29] Nonetheless, given the implications of a further event, this decision should be discussed with the woman and her view taken into account. Graduated elastic compression stockings and/or low-dose aspirin can be employed antenatally in these women. Postpartum pharmacological prophylaxis, with or without graduated elastic compression stockings, should be given for at least 6 weeks. If treatment is switched to warfarin postpartum the target international normalised ratio (INR) is 2–3 and LMWH should be continued until the INR is 2.0.

In women with a single previous VTE and underlying thrombophilia, previous idiopathic VTE or additional risk factors such as obesity, the case for antenatal pharmacological prophylaxis is much stronger. Antenatally, these women should be considered for prophylactic LMWH with or without graduated elastic compression stockings. In the presence of antithrombin deficiency more intense LMWH therapy is usually prescribed, although many such women will already be on long-term anticoagulant therapy. Postpartum pharmacological thromboprophylaxis, with or without graduated elastic compression stockings, for at least 6 weeks is recommended.

Multiple previous VTE

Women with multiple previous VTE should receive antenatal LMWH thromboprophylaxis and wear graduated elastic compression stockings. Postpartum pharmacological thromboprophylaxis, with or without graduated elastic compression stockings, for at least 6 weeks is recommended. A higher dose of antenatal LMWH and longer duration of postpartum prophylaxis may be required for women with additional risk factors.

Women with previous VTE on long-term anticoagulants should switch from oral anticoagulants to treatment doses of LMWH by 6 weeks of gestation, and should be fitted with graduated elastic compression stockings. Postpartum, long-term anticoagulants, with LMWH overlap until the INR reaches prepregnancy therapeutic levels, should be resumed.

Known thrombophilia without VTE

Where a woman without prior VTE is known to have a heritable thrombophilia, either surveillance or prophylactic LMWH with or without graduated elastic compression stockings can be used antenatally. In women who are antithrombin deficient and in strongly symptomatic kindred there is a strong case for antenatal LMWH. Postpartum pharmacological thromboprophylaxis, with or without graduated elastic compression stockings, for at least 6 weeks is recommended.

RECOMMENDATIONS FOR GYNAECOLOGICAL SURGERY

Pharmacological prophylaxis with heparin, LMWH, warfarin and dextran, and mechanical methods such as graduated elastic compression stockings

---

Table 7.4 Risk assessment profile for thromboembolism in gynaecological surgery

LOW RISK – Early mobilisation and hydration

Minor surgery (<30 min); no other risk factors
Major surgery (<30 min); age <40 years and no other risk factors

MODERATE RISK –
Consider one of a variety of prophylactic measures available

Minor surgery (<30 min) in patients with a personal or family history of deep-vein thrombosis, pulmonary embolism or thrombophilia
Major surgery (>30 min)
Laparoscopic extended surgery
Obesity (>80 kg)
Gross varicose veins
Current infection
Immobility prior to surgery (>4 days)
Major current illness, e.g. heart or lung disease; inflammatory bowel disease; nephrotic syndrome; malignancies (other than gynaecological)
Heart failure or recent myocardial infarction

HIGH RISK – Heparin prophylaxis +/- compression stockings

A total of three or more moderate-risk factors above
Major pelvic or abdominal surgery for gynaecological cancer
Major surgery (>30 min) in patients with:
    a personal or family history of previous deep-vein thrombosis, pulmonary embolism
    thrombophilia
    paralysis or immobilisation of lower limbs

modified from RCOG[5]

---

and pneumatic calf compression are effective in preventing postoperative thromboembolism. Their use has been emphasised in consensus documents from the UK in 2002[1] and North America in 2004.[30]

Women undergoing gynaecological surgery should be assessed for clinical risk factors (Table 7.4) and the need for thromboprophylaxis based on the degree of risk. Individual clinicians and units should develop clear policies for thromboprophylaxis. Current recommended practice is as follows:

- Women at low risk should be encouraged to mobilise early and avoid dehydration in the postoperative period.
- Women at moderate risk, in addition to early mobilisation and avoidance of postoperative dehydration, should receive pharmacological prophylaxis, commencing before surgery and continuing until discharge from hospital. Low-dose UFH 5 000 iu 12-hourly or subcutaneous LMWH (e.g. enoxaparin 20 mg/day or dalteparin 2 500 iu/day) is recommended.[1,5] Graduated elastic compression stockings and intermittent calf compression are an alternative in women for whom heparin is contraindicated.
- Women at high risk should be managed as for women with a moderate risk, but larger doses of subcutaneous UFH (5 000 iu 8 hourly) or subcutaneous LMWH (e.g. enoxaparin 40 mg/day or dalteparin 5 000 iu/day) should be used, and combined with mechanical methods. Prophylaxis should continue at least until discharge from hospital and continuation following discharge must be considered.

Diagnosis of VTE

The symptoms and signs of DVT include leg pain, swelling, tenderness, oedema, pyrexia, lower abdominal pain and elevated white cell count. Pulmonary embolus may present with chest pain, dyspnoea, haemoptysis, collapse, raised jugular venous pressure, focal signs in the chest and symptoms and signs of DVT. However, the clinical diagnosis of VTE is unreliable, particularly in pregnancy, where leg swelling and discomfort are common features.[31] Objective diagnosis of VTE in pregnancy is essential, as failure to identify a VTE will endanger the mother, while unnecessary treatment will expose her to the hazards of therapeutic anticoagulation. Such treatment may also label her as having had a VTE, a factor that will significantly alter her future health care with regard to contraception, thromboprophylaxis in future pregnancies, and hormone replacement therapy in later life.

Real-time or duplex ultrasound venography is the main diagnostic tool for DVT.[32] A negative ultrasound report with a low level of clinical suspicion suggests that anticoagulant treatment can be discontinued or withheld. Where there is a negative ultrasound and high clinical suspicion, anticoagulation should be continued and ultrasound repeated in one week, or alternative imaging techniques such as X-ray venography or MRI considered. If repeat testing is negative, anticoagulant treatment should be discontinued.[33]

If PTE is suspected both a ventilation/perfusion (V/Q) lung scan and bilateral duplex ultrasound leg examinations should be performed. In the nonpregnant, a normal perfusion scan has a negative predictive value of over 99% and a high probability lung scan has a positive predictive value of over 85%. Where there is strong clinical suspicion of PTE the positive predictive value of a high probability lung scan increases to over 95% but with low clinical suspicion probability decreases to less than 60%. The greatest diagnostic problem is when the V/Q scan is in the medium range. In practical terms when the V/Q scan reports a 'medium' or 'high' probability of PTE or there is 'low' probability of PTE on V/Q scan but positive ultrasound for DVT, anticoagulant treatment should be continued. When a V/Q scan reports a low risk of PTE and there are negative leg ultrasound examinations, yet high clinical suspicion, anticoagulant treatment should continue with repeat testing in one week (V/Q scan and leg ultrasound examination) or alternative imaging techniques such as pulmonary angiography or magnetic resonance imaging or helical computerised tomography should be employed.[33]

Helical computed tomography (CT) scanning is of value and can rapidly image the whole thorax with good visualisation to the level of the segmental arteries. Echocardiography, particularly when performed trans-oesophageally, may allow direct visualisation of thrombus in the pulmonary arteries or right heart. Indirect signs of PTE include a dilated hypokinetic right ventricle, tricuspid regurgitation and high pulmonary artery pressures as measured with Doppler ultrasound.

The radiation dose from investigations such as V/Q scanning, chest X-ray, helical CT and even limited venography is modest[34] and considered to pose a negligible risk to the fetus particularly when set in the context of the risk from PTE. It must be emphasised that objective diagnostic testing should not be withheld during pregnancy because of concern regarding fetal radiation exposure.

D-dimer is used as a screening test for VTE in the nonpregnant where it has a high negative predictive value: a low level of D-dimer suggests the absence of VTE and further objective tests are not performed, while an increased level of D-dimer leads to an objective diagnostic test for VTE.[32] In pregnancy D-dimer can be increased owing to the physiological changes in the coagulation system and also if there is a concomitant problem such as pre-eclampsia. Thus, a 'positive' D-dimer test in pregnancy is not necessarily consistent with VTE and objective diagnostic testing is required. However, a low level of D-dimer in pregnancy is likely, as in the nonpregnant, to suggest that there is no VTE. Nonetheless there is limited information on D-dimer screening for VTE in pregnancy and firm guidance cannot be given.

Thrombophilia screening (see Chapter 8) at the time of presentation and before starting anticoagulant therapy may occasionally be useful in women with VTE. Although the result may be influenced by pregnancy or thrombus and will not influence immediate management, it may influence the duration and intensity of anticoagulation, for example if antithrombin deficiency is identified. It is important that clinicians with specific expertise interpret the results of any thrombophilia screen performed.

Management of acute VTE

When DVT or PTE are suspected clinically, treatment with UFH or LMWH should be given until the diagnosis is excluded by objective testing, unless anticoagulation is contraindicated. Graduated elastic compression stockings and leg elevation should be employed for DVT. Analgesia for pleuritic pain and oxygen are often required in PTE.

Traditionally, UFH has been used in the initial management of VTE as such treatment reduces the risk of further thromboembolism compared with no treatment. UFH is preferred to LMWH by some authorities in the initial management of massive PTE because of its rapid effect and because of traditional experience of this drug.

UFH can be given by continuous intravenous infusion. Subcutaneous UFH (15 000–20 000 iu, 12-hourly after an initial intravenous bolus of 5000 iu) is an effective alternative.[35] The dose of UFH is adjusted by monitoring the APTT with a therapeutic target ratio of 1.5–2.5 times the mean laboratory control value.[36] The APTT should be performed 6 hours after the loading dose then daily. Failure to achieve the lower limit of the target APTT therapeutic range carries a 10–15-fold increase in the risk of recurrent VTE.[37] APTT may be technically problematic, particularly in late pregnancy when apparent heparin resistance occurs because of increased fibrinogen and factor VIII. This can lead to unnecessarily high doses of heparin being used with subsequent haemorrhagic problems. Where such problems exist, anti-Xa levels may be useful as a measure of heparin dose (target range 0.35–0.7 iu/ml).

In nonpregnant patients, LMWH is as effective as UFH and is associated with lower mortality and lower risk of haemorrhagic complications in the initial treatment of DVT.[38,39] LMWH is as effective as UFH in the initial treatment of PTE.[40] LMWH has been recommended for the initial management of VTE in pregnancy.[16,41]

In nonpregnant patients, once daily administration is recommended for acute treatment of VTE with LMWH. In view of altered pharmacokinetics in pregnancy, a twice-daily regimen is recommended for the LMWHs

Table 7.5 The initial dose of enoxaparin for acute treatment of VTE is determined by body weight

Early pregnancy weight	Initial dose of enoxaparin
<50 kg	40 mg twice daily
50–69 kg	60 mg twice daily
70–89 kg	80 mg twice daily
≤90 kg	100 mg twice daily

dalteparin and enoxaparin in the treatment of VTE in pregnancy. One regimen for the administration of LMWH (enoxaparin) in the immediate management of VTE in pregnancy is shown in Table 7.5. The dose closest to the woman's early pregnancy weight should be employed and continued 12 hourly until objective testing has been performed. If the diagnosis of VTE is confirmed treatment is continued. Peak anti-Xa activity (three hours post-injection) can be measured to confirm that an appropriate dose has been given. If the level is above the upper limit of the therapeutic target range (0.6–1.2 iu/ml) the dose of LMWH should be reduced and peak anti-Xa activity reassessed. Satisfactory anti-Xa levels are obtained using this regimen and further monitoring of anti-Xa levels can be deferred until the next routine working day.[41] It is important to prescribe an adequate dose of heparin in women with a high BMI.[2]

A temporary vena cava filter may be required in recurrent PTE despite satisfactory anticoagulation or where anticoagulation is contraindicated.[42] Thrombolytic therapy may be necessary for life-threatening PTE or where massive DVT threatens limb viability. Experience is limited and there is a risk of major haemorrhage if systemic thrombolysis is used around the time of delivery or postpartum. Percutaneous catheter thrombus fragmentation or surgical embolectomy are alternative measures if local expertise is available.[42]

With heparin therapy, the platelet count should be monitored 4–8 days after treatment commences, then monthly to detect heparin-induced thrombocytopenia. Pregnant women who develop heparin-induced thrombocytopenia and require continuing anticoagulant therapy can be managed with the heparinoid danaparoid sodium,[43] or if postpartum, treated with warfarin.

Subcutaneous LMWH is usually used for maintenance treatment of VTE for the remainder of pregnancy.[41] Therapeutic doses should be employed for maintenance therapy, as a high recurrence rate of VTE has been reported in nonpregnant patients receiving thromboprophylactic maintenance doses of UFH.[44] Women can be taught to self-inject and can be managed as outpatients once the acute event has been dealt with. Arrangements should be made for safe disposal of needles and syringes. Outpatient follow-up should include assessment of platelet and peak anti-Xa levels.

The duration of therapeutic anticoagulant treatment in nonpregnant patients is usually 6 months. As pregnancy is associated with prothrombotic changes in the coagulation system and venous flow it seems logical to apply this duration of therapy to pregnancy. If the VTE occurs early in pregnancy then, provided that there are no additional risk factors, the dose of LMWH could be reduced after 6 months to prophylactic levels (40 mg enoxaparin or 5000 iu dalteparin once per day). Following delivery treatment should continue for at least 6–12 weeks. If the woman chooses to commence warfarin postpartum, this can usually be initiated on the second or third postnatal day. The INR should be checked on day two and subsequent warfarin doses titrated to maintain the INR between 2.0–3.0.[45] Heparin should be continued until the INR is >2.0 on two successive days.

LABOUR AND DELIVERY IN WOMEN ON ANTICOAGULANT THERAPY

The woman on anticoagulants should be advised that once she thinks that she may be in labour, she should not inject heparin until she has been assessed and that medical staff should prescribe any further doses. Where induction of labour is planned the dose of heparin should be reduced to its thromboprophylactic dose on the day prior to delivery, and the treatment dose (twice-daily administration) recommenced following delivery.

Epidural anaesthesia should be sited only after discussion with a senior anaesthetist because of the small risk of epidural haematoma formation during spinal instrumentation in anticoagulated patients. If used, extra vigilance for signs of cord compression should be maintained. The timing of anaesthesia and/or heparin administration needs to be coordinated. Generally, regional techniques are not used until at least 12 hours after the previous prophylactic dose of LMWH. When a woman presents on a therapeutic regimen of LMWH, regional techniques should not be employed for at least 24 hours after the last dose of LMWH. LMWH should not be given for at least 3 hours after the epidural catheter has been removed and the cannula should not be removed within 10–12 hours of the most recent injection.[46,47]

For elective caesarean section, the woman should receive a thromboprophylactic dose of LMWH on the day before delivery. On the day of delivery the morning dose should be omitted and the operation performed as soon as possible thereafter. Graduated elastic compression stockings or mechanical methods may be used to provide intraoperative prophylaxis. A thromboprophylactic dose of LMWH should be given by three hours postoperatively and after removal of the epidural catheter. The treatment dose should be recommenced that evening. This reflects general principles – individual management plans are often required with regard to anticoagulant treatment. The risk of wound haematoma following caesarean section is around 2% with both UFH and LMWH. Use of drains (abdominal and rectus sheath) should be considered, and the skin incision closed with staples or interrupted sutures to allow drainage of any haematoma.

If continued heparin treatment is considered essential in a woman considered to be at high risk of haemorrhage, for example because of recent major haemorrhage or coagulopathy, suspected intra-abdominal bleeding or progressive wound haematoma, intravenous UFH should be given until the risk factors for haemorrhage have resolved. This is because intravenous UFH is short acting and anticoagulation will reverse soon after cessation of the infusion should a haemorrhagic problem occur.

Gynaecological surgery and women on the oral contraceptive pill or postmenopausal hormone replacement therapy

Controversy surrounds the use of the combined oral contraceptive pill in women undergoing major surgery,[48,49] because it is associated with changes in the coagulation system. Briefly, an increase in procoagulants, including factors VII and X and fibrinogen, occur together with a reduction in concentrations of antithrombin. However, there is also an increase in fibrinolysis, which may balance the procoagulant changes. The effects are oestrogen related, with pills containing lower doses of oestrogen showing the least change in haemostatic factors. The changes are also modified by the progestogen component of the pill. From an epidemiological perspective, clear evidence from case–control studies links the combined pill with VTE. However, factors such as underlying congenital thrombophilia have not yet been taken into account. It is important when prescribing the pill to consider such risk factors but there is minimal information with regard to postoperative VTE.

The risk of postoperative VTE increases from 0.5% to 1% for pill users compared with nonusers.[50] This small excess risk in pill users must be balanced against the risks of stopping the pill 4–6 weeks prior to surgery, including unwanted pregnancy, effects of surgery and anaesthesia on a pregnancy, and risks of subsequent termination. Therefore, this decision should, after full discussion, be tailored on an individual basis for each woman and clinical situation. Risks should be communicated to the woman and, if agreed, adequate alternative contraception should be arranged until combined oral contraceptives are restarted. The timing of restarting combined oral contraceptives will involve individual assessment, for example of postoperative complications or immobility. When considering perioperative prophylaxis in current (or within past month) pill users, each case should be judged according to additional risk factors.[1] In emergency surgery, VTE prophylaxis should be given routinely as the risk of VTE is greater.

PROGESTOGEN-ONLY CONTRACEPTIVES

There is no evidence that low doses of progestogens used for contraception are associated with increased risk of VTE, or should be stopped prior to elective surgery. They may be an alternative for women at high risk of VTE stopping their combined oral contraceptive pill.[51] There is, however, evidence of an increase of five- to six-fold in VTE risk with higher doses of progestogen used for other therapeutic indications (e.g. menstrual disorders).[52,53]

HORMONE REPLACEMENT THERAPY AND RALOXIFENE

Oral oestrogen-containing hormone replacement therapy (HRT), and the selective oestrogen receptor modulator, raloxifene,[54] increase the risk of VTE three-fold, especially in the first year of use. This translates to an absolute risk of 30 per 100 000 women per year for users of HRT compared with 10 per 100 000 women per year for nonusers. Women wishing to continue HRT in the presence of additional clinical risk factors should be referred to a specialist with expertise in thrombophilia.[1] Transdermal HRT may be preferred in such women because it has a lesser effect on haemostasis than oral HRT.[55]

Summary

VTE remains the major cause of mortality in association with pregnancy and childbirth and a source of morbidity that continues into later life. VTE impacts significantly upon postoperative morbidity and mortality in gynaecological surgery. If the incidence and consequences of VTE are to be significantly reduced, obstetricians and gynaecologists must understand the risk factors for VTE, the appropriate use of prophylaxis particularly after vaginal delivery, the need for objective diagnosis in women with suspected VTE and the principles of anticoagulant therapy.

Key points

- Venous thromboembolism is common and is a significant cause of death in hospital patients, the leading cause of direct maternal death in the UK, and frequently results in longterm problems for survivors.
- Thromboprophylaxis is effective in reducing the incidence of VTE.
- Women undergoing gynaecological surgery should be assessed for clinical risk and appropriate thromboprophylaxis should be prescribed.
- The risk of VTE should be assessed early in all pregnant women and reviewed if new risk factors arise. Appropriate thromboprophylaxis should be prescribed.
- Air and other forms of long-distance travel increases the risk of VTE. Pregnant women planning to travel should be given specific advice.
- Graduated compression stockings are recommended for hospital inpatients at increased risk of VTE.
- Women with previous VTE should be screened for inherited and acquired thrombophilia.
- Age over 35 years and BMI >30 are important independent risk factors for VTE even after vaginal delivery. Women at moderately increased risk (two risk factors) should have postpartum thromboprophylaxis with LMWH for 3–5 days.
- In pregnancy, women with previous recurrent VTE, or previous VTE and first-degree family history of VTE, or previous VTE and thrombophilia should receive antenatal thromboprophylaxis with LMWH, and postpartum thromboprophylaxis for 6 weeks.
- Warfarin should be avoided in pregnancy. It crosses the placenta, is teratogenic and may cause fetal haemorrhage.
- Heparin does not cross the placenta. LMWH is the anticoagulant of choice for antenatal thromboprophylaxis as it is effective and safer than unfractionated heparin.
- The platelet count should be monitored monthly in women receiving long-term UFH or LMWH.
- Aspirin is effective in surgical patients and may be useful for long-term thromboprophylaxis after discharge from hospital, or when other thromboprophylactic measures are unsuitable or contraindicated, or during pregnancy where there is an increased risk of VTE but uncertainty whether LMWH is justified.
- At least 12 hours (24 hours for therapeutic doses) should elapse between the last prophylactic dose of LMWH and the introduction or removal of a spinal or epidural catheter.

continued on following page

continued from previous page

- Anticoagulants are not contraindicated for breastfeeding mothers as neither heparin nor warfarin is secreted in significant amounts in breast milk.
- The clinical diagnosis of VTE is unreliable. If there is clinical suspicion of VTE, treatment with intravenous or subcutaneous unfractionated heparin or LMWH should be given until the diagnosis is excluded by objective testing.
- Real-time or duplex venography is the main method of diagnosing DVT, and if PTE is suspected, a ventilation/perfusion lung scan should also be performed.
- Radiological investigations to diagnose VTE during pregnancy do not pose a significant risk to the fetus.
- A low level of D-dimer suggests that there is no VTE.
- LMWHs are as effective as and have fewer complications than unfractionated heparin for the initial treatment of VTE.
- Women taking anticoagulants during pregnancy should be advised not to administer any further doses if they think labour has started.
- There is a small increased risk of VTE in women taking the combined oral contraceptive pill or hormone replacement therapy. For elective surgery, discontinuing treatment should be discussed with the woman on an individual basis, and thromboprophylaxis considered; for emergency surgery, routine thromboprophylaxis should be given.

References

1 Scottish Intercollegiate Guidelines Network. *Prophylaxis of Venous Thromboembolism*. Edinburgh: SIGN; 2002.

2 Drife J. Thrombosis and thromboembolism. In: Lewis G, Drife J, editors. *Why Mothers Die 2000–2002. The Sixth Report of Confidential Enquiries into Maternal Deaths in the United Kingdom*. London: RCOG Press; 2004. p 61–78.

3 McColl MD, Ellison J, Greer IA, Tait RC, Walker ID. Prevalence of the post-thrombotic syndrome in young women with previous venous thromboembolism. *Br J Haematol* 2000;108(2):272–4.

4 Macklon NS, Greer IA. Venous thromboembolic disease in obstetrics and gynaecology: the Scottish experience. *Scot Med J* 1996;41:83–6.

5 Royal College of Obstetricians and Gynaecologists. *Report of the RCOG Working Party on Prophylaxis against Thromboembolism in Gynaecology and Obstetrics*. London: RCOG; 1995.

6   Geerts WH, Heit JA, Clagett GP, *et al.* Prevention of venous thromboembolism. *Chest* 2001;119(Suppl 1):132S–175S.

7   Macklon NS, Greer IA, Bowman AW. An ultrasound study of gestational and postural changes in the deep venous system of the leg in pregnancy. *Br J Obstet Gynaecol* 1997;104(2):191–7.

8   McColl MD, Ramsay JE, Tait RC, *et al.* Risk factors for pregnancy associated venous thromboembolism. *Thromb Haemost* 1997;78(4):1183–8.

9   Flessa HC, Kapstrom AB, Glueck HI, Will JJ. Placental transport of heparin. *Am J Obstet Gynecol* 1965;93(4):570–73.

10 Forestier F, Daffos F, Capella-Pavlovsky M. Low molecular weight heparin (PK 10169) does not cross the placenta during the second trimester of pregnancy study by direct fetal blood sampling under ultrasound. *Thromb Res* 1984;34(6):557–60.

11 Forestier F, Daffos F, Rainaut M, Toulemonde F. Low molecular weight heparin (CY 216) does not cross the placenta during the third trimester of pregnancy. *Thromb Haemost* 1987;57(2):234.

12 Sanson BJ, Lensing AW, Prins MH, et al. Safety of low-molecular-weight heparin in pregnancy: a systematic review. *Thromb Haemost* 1999;81(5):668–72.

13 Nelson-Piercy C. Hazards of heparin: allergy, heparin-induced thrombo-cytopenia and osteoporosis. *Baillière's Clin Obstet Gynaecol* 1997;11(3):489–509.

14 Pettila V, Leinonen P, Markkola A, Hiilesmaa V, Kaaja R. Postpartum bone mineral density in women treated for thromboprophylaxis with unfractionated heparin or LMW heparin. *Thromb Haemost* 2002;87(2):182–6.

15 Warkentin TE, Levine MN, Hirsh J, *et al.* Heparin-induced thrombocytopenia in patients treated with low-molecular-weight heparin or unfractionated heparin. *N Engl J Med* 1995;332(20):1330–35.

16 Greer IA, Hunt B. Low molecular weight heparin in pregnancy: current issues. *Br J Haematol* 2004;128:593–601.

17 Bates SM, Ginsberg JS. Anticoagulants in pregnancy: fetal defects. In: Greer IA, editor. *Baillière's Clin Obstet Gynaecol* 1997;11(3):479–88.

18 Vitale N, De Feo M, De Santo LS, Pollice A, Tedesco N, Cotrufo M. Dose-dependent fetal complications of warfarin in pregnant women with mechanical heart valves. *J Am Coll Cardiol* 1999;33(6):1637–41.

19 Letsky E. Peripartum prophylaxis of thromboembolism. In: Greer IA, editor. *Baillière's Clin Obstet Gynaecol* 1997;11(3):523–43.

20 Poller L, McKernan A, Thomson JM, Elstein M, Hirsch PJ, Jones JB. Fixed minidose warfarin: a new approach to prophylaxis against venous thrombosis after major surgery. *BMJ* 1987;295(6609):1309–12.

21 Gruber UF, Saldeen T, Brokop T, *et al.* Incidences of fatal postoperative pulmonary embolism after prophylaxis with dextran 70 and low-dose heparin: an international multicentre study. *BMJ* 1980;280(6207):69–72.

22 Barbier P, Jonville AP, Autret E, Coureau C. Fetal risks with dextrans during delivery. *Drug Saf* 1992;7(1):71–3.

23 Clagett GP, Anderson FA, Geerts W, *et al.* Prevention of venous thrombo-embolism. *Chest* 1998;114(suppl 5):531S–560S.

24 Imperiale TF, Petrulis AS. A meta-analysis of low-dose aspirin for the prevention of pregnancy-induced hypertensive disease. *JAMA* 1991;266(2):260–64.

25 CLASP (Collaborative Low-dose Aspirin Study in Pregnancy) Collaborative Group. CLASP: a randomised trial of low-dose aspirin for the prevention and treatment of pre-eclampsia among 9364 pregnant women. *Lancet* 1994;343(8898):619–29.

26 Lindhoff-Last EWA, Thalhammer C, Nowak G, Bauersachs R. Hirudin treatment in a breastfeeding woman. *Lancet* 2000;355(9202):467–8.

27 Macklon NS, Greer IA. Technical note: compression stockings and posture: a comparative study of their effects on the proximal deep veins of the leg at rest. *Br J Radiol* 1995;68(809):515–8.

28 Royal College of Obstetricians and Gynaecologists. *Advice on Preventing Deep Vein Thrombosis for Pregnant Women Travelling by Air.* Scientific Advisory Committee Opinion Paper 1. London: RCOG; 2001.

29 Brill-Edwards P, Ginsberg JS, Gent M, *et al.* Safety of withholding heparin in pregnant women with a history of venous thromboembolism. Recurrence of Clot in This Pregnancy Study Group. *N Engl J Med* 2000;343(20):1439–44.

30 ACCP. Seventh ACCP Consensus Conference on Antithrombotic Therapy. *Chest* 2004;126(3 Suppl):1–644S.

31 Bates SM, Greer IA, Hirsh J, Ginsberg JS. Use of antithrombotic agents during pregnancy: the Seventh ACCP Conference on Antithrombotic and Thrombolytic Therapy. *Chest* 2004;126(3 Suppl):627–44S.

32 Macklon NS. Diagnosis of deep venous thrombosis and pulmonary embolism. In: Greer IA, editor. *Baillière's Clin Obstet Gynaecol* 1997;11(3):463–77.

33 Thomson AJ, Greer IA. Emergencies in obstetrics and gynaecology: non-haemorrhagic obstetric shock. *Baillière's Clin Obstet Gynaecol* 2000;14:19–41.

34 Ginsberg JS, Hirsh J, Rainbow AJ, Coates G. Risks to the fetus of radiologic procedures used in the diagnosis of maternal venous thromboembolic disease. *Thromb Haemost* 1989;61(2):189–96.

35 Hommes DW, Bura A, Mazzolai L, Buller HR, ten Cate JW. Subcutaneous heparin compared with continuous intravenous heparin administration in the initial treatment of deep vein thrombosis. A meta-analysis. *Ann Intern Med* 1992;116(4):279–84.

36 Lowe GD. Treatment of venous thrombo-embolism. *Baillière's Clin Obstet Gynaecol* 1997;11(3):511–21.

37 Hyers TM, Hull RD, Weg JG. Antithrombotic therapy for venous thromboembolic disease. *Chest* 1995;108(suppl 4):335S–351S.

38 Dolovich L, Ginsberg JS. Low molecular weight heparin in the treatment of venous thromboembolism: an updated meta-analysis. *Vessels* 1997;3:4–11.

39 Gould MK, Dembitzer AD, Doyle RL, Hastie TJ, Garber AM. Low-molecular-weight heparins compared with unfractionated heparin for treatment of acute deep venous thrombosis. A meta-analysis of randomized, controlled trials. *Ann Intern Med* 1999;130(10):800–809.

40 Simonneau G, Sors H, Charbonnier B, Page Y, Laaban JP, Azarian R *et al.* A comparison of low-molecular-weight heparin with unfractionated heparin for acute pulmonary embolism. The THESEE Study Group. Tinzaparine ou Heparine Standard: Evaluations dans l'Embolie Pulmonaire. *N Engl J Med* 1997;337(10):663–9.

41 Thomson A, Walker I, Greer I. Low-molecular-weight heparin for immediate management of thromboembolic disease in pregnancy. *Lancet* 1998;352:1904.

42 Royal College of Obstetricians and Gynaecologists. *Thromboembolic Disease in Pregnancy and the Puerperium: Acute Management.* Guideline No. 28. London: RCOG; 2001.

43 Magnani HN. Heparin-induced thrombocytopenia (HIT): an overview of 230 patients treated with orgaran (Org 10172) [published erratum appears in *Thromb Haemost* 1993 Dec 20;70(6):1072]. *Thromb Haemost* 1993;70(4):554–61.

44 Hull R, Delmore T, Carter C, *et al.* Adjusted subcutaneous heparin versus warfarin sodium in the long-term treatment of venous thrombosis. *N Engl J Med* 1982;306(4):189–94.

45 Haemostasis and Thrombosis Task Force. Guidelines on oral anticoagulation: third edition. *Br J Haematol* 1998;101(2):374–87.

46 Horlocker TT, Wedel DJ. Spinal and epidural blockade and perioperative low molecular weight heparin: smooth sailing on the Titanic. *Anesth Analg* 1998;86(6):1153–6.

47 Checketts MR, Wildsmith JA. Central nerve block and thromboprophylaxis – is there a problem? *Br J Anaesth* 1999;82(2):164–7.

48 Guillebaud J. Surgery and the pill. *BMJ* 1985;291(6494):498–9.

49 Sue-Ling H, Hughes LE. Should the pill be stopped preoperatively? *BMJ* 1988; 296(6620):447–8.

50 Vessey MP, Doll R, Fairbairn AS, Glober G. Postoperative thromboembolism and the use of oral contraceptives. *BMJ* 1970;3(715):123–6.

51 British Committee for Standards in Haematology (BCSH). Investigation and management of heritable thrombophilia. Haemostasis and Thrombosis Task Force. *Br J Haematol* 2001;114(3):512–28.

52 Poulter NR, Chang CL, Farley TM, Meirik O. Risk of cardiovascular diseases associated with oral progestagen preparations with therapeutic indications. *Lancet* 1999;354(9190):1610.

53 Vasilakis C, Jick H, del Mar, Melero-Montes M. Risk of idiopathic venous thrombo-embolism in users of progestagens alone. *Lancet* 1999;354(9190):1610–11.

54 Ettinger B, Black DM, Mitlak BH, *et al.* Reduction of vertebral fracture risk in postmenopausal women with osteoporosis treated with raloxifene: results from a 3-year randomized clinical trial. Multiple Outcomes of Raloxifene Evaluation (MORE) Investigators. *JAMA* 1999;282(7):637–45.

55 Lowe GD, Upton MN, Rumley A, McConnachie A, O'Reilly DS, Watt GC. Different effects of oral and transdermal hormone replacement therapies on factor IX, APC resistance, t-PA, PAI and C-reactive protein – a cross-sectional population survey. *Thromb Haemost* 2001;86(2):550–56.

56 Scottish Intercollegiate Guidelines Network. *Prophylaxis of Venous Thromboembolism.* Edinburgh: SIGN; 1995.

8 Genetic thrombophilias and antiphospholipid antibodies

The term 'thrombophilia' defines situations associated with an increased risk of venous thromboembolism (VTE) characterised by hypercoagulability. Normal haemostasis requires the maintenance of a balance between the procoagulant system, which provides protection from bleeding after vascular injury, and the anticoagulant system, which protects against the effects of excessive coagulation (see Chapter 1). Overactivity in procoagulant factors or underactivity in anticoagulant factors may upset this balance, resulting in a predisposition to VTE. Changes in the circulating levels of pro- and anticoagulant proteins, venous blood flow and the vascular endothelium all contribute to the hypercoaguable state associated with normal pregnancy. Some individuals also have a genetic or acquired thrombophilia. Thrombosis and thrombophilia have been implicated in the pathophysiology of a number of obstetric complications including recurrent miscarriage, intrauterine growth restriction, placental abruption and pre-eclampsia.

Molecular risk factors for VTE may be genetic or phenotypic. Genetic factors comprise all mutations responsible for a loss or gain of function that predispose to VTE such as deficiencies of the naturally occurring anticoagulants and genetic mutations of factor V and prothrombin. Phenotypic factors are abnormalities in laboratory tests that are associated with VTE and may have both genetic and environmental influences.

Exploration of the pathogenesis of VTE has produced a multifactorial model of disease that depends on variable combinations of acquired and genetic risk factors (Table 8.1). Familial clustering of cases illustrates the genetic component, while the episodic nature of events implicates an acquired or environmental influence. It is estimated that genetic factors play a role in up to 50% of people with VTE.

This chapter provides an overview of the more common genetic thrombophilias and the acquired thrombophilia associated with the presence of antiphospholipid antibodies. Several reviews elaborate on the material presented in this chapter.[1–8]

Table 8.1 Risk factors for venous thromboembolism (VTE)

Persistent			Transient
Inherited	**Acquired**	**Mixed or not well established**	
Antithrombin III deficiency	Age	Hyperhomo-cysteinaemia	Surgery
Protein C deficiency	Malignancy	High factor VIII	Major trauma
Protein S deficiency	Antiphospholipid antibodies	High factor IX	Pregnancy and puerperium
Factor V Leiden	History of VTE	High factor XI	OCP/HRT
Prothrombin G20210A	Myeloproliferative disorders	High TAFI	Prolonged immobilisation
		Protein C resistance (without factor V Leiden) Dysfibrinogenaemia High fibrinogen	

OCP = oral contraceptive HRT = hormone replacement therapy
TAFI = thrombin activatable fibrinolysis inhibitor

Genetic thrombophilia

A limited number of genetic variants are proven to be independent risk factors for VTE. These include mutations in the genes controlling the function of both pro- and anticoagulant factors. Mutations may result in a quantitative (type 1) or qualitative (type 2) defect in protein function.

DEFICIENCIES OF THE NATURALLY OCCURRING ANTICOAGULANTS

Mutations have been identified in the genes encoding the major naturally occurring anticoagulants antithrombin, protein C and protein S. Homozygous deficiencies of protein C or protein S lead to severe thrombotic manifestations such as neonatal purpura fulminans and warfarin-induced skin necrosis. No homozygous antithrombin deficiencies have been reported. In general heterozygous deficiencies of naturally occurring anticoagulants lead to thrombosis at an early age, often without environmental triggers, and sometimes in unusual sites. These individuals have a tendency to recurrent VTE and often have a family history of it. The frequency of deficiencies of naturally occurring anticoagulants in the general population is low (<1%). They are transmitted in an autosomal dominant fashion, and occur in about 5–10% of people with thrombosis.

Antithrombin
Antithrombin (AT) is the most powerful of the naturally occurring anticoagulants, inhibiting the action not only of thrombin, but also of the activated clotting factors IXa, Xa, XIIa and tissue-bound factor VIIa. More than 75 different mutations in the AT gene have been identified. Heterozygosity for AT deficiency confers a five-fold increase in risk of VTE.

Protein C
Protein C (PC) is activated by the thrombin-thrombomodulin complex. Activated protein C (aPC) degrades the activated clotting factors Va and VIIIa. The inhibitory effects of PC are facilitated through the cofactor activity of protein S. More than 160 PC gene mutations have been identified. Heterozygosity for PC deficiency confers a seven-fold increase in risk of VTE.

Protein S
Protein S (PS) is the nonenzymatic cofactor of aPC in the inactivation of factors Va and VIIa, but also has aPC-independent anticoagulant activity. PS exists in free (40%) and bound (60%) forms, and it is only the former that has anticoagulant activity. Free PS measurements are better able to distinguish heterozygous PS-deficient subjects from normal individuals. PS gene mutations not infrequently occur with the factor V Leiden (FVL) mutation, conferring an increased risk of VTE at an earlier age. Around 70 different PS mutations have been described; heterozygosity results in a six- to ten-fold increase in risk of VTE.

GAIN OF FUNCTION MUTATIONS

Factor V Leiden and the prothrombin G20210A mutation both give rise to protein overactivity. These mutations are found at a relatively high frequency among Western populations, and expression of both mutations is not uncommon. Dual expression is associated with a higher risk of VTE than either mutation alone.

Factor V Leiden
Factor V Leiden is the most common cause of thombophilia (up to 50% of people with VTE). A mutation in the factor V gene results in an abnormal factor V protein that is resistant to the action of aPC. The mutation is relatively common in those of European descent (2–15%). Heterozygotes have a seven-fold increase in risk of VTE, while homozygotes have an

eighty-fold increase in risk. Carriers often have mild thrombotic manifest-ations and may present at a relatively advanced age. There are strong interactions with PC, PS and prothrombin G20210A mutations. The aPC resistance phenotype may also occur in the absence of the FVL mutation. Other specific mutations may be responsible but environmental influences may also be important. Pregnancy produces aPC resistance as the result of increased levels of factor V and factor VIII; the oral contraceptives and antiphospholipid antibodies can also confer aPC resistance.

Prothrombin G20210A

The prothrombin G20210A mutation produces a prothrombin molecule that persists in the circulation for longer than usual, increasing the circulating level of prothrombin and the potential for thrombosis. The mutation occurs in 2–4% of the white population, and in around 20% of people with VTE. Heterozygotes have a two- to four-fold higher risk of VTE than noncarriers.

OTHER PHENOTYPES

The role of the following factors in producing VTE is less well established; their levels may be genetically determined, but may also be substantially influenced by environmental factors.

Hyperhomocysteinaemia

Hyperhomocysteinaemia is associated with an increased risk of both venous and arterial thrombosis of the order of two- to three-fold. The biochemical abnormality is commonly the result of homozygosity for the thermolabile variant of methylenetetrahydrofolate reductase (MTHFR), which occurs in about 11% of the UK population. However, an association between this genetic marker and the risk of VTE has not been demonstrated, possibly because folate deficiency is a prerequisite for the development of hyperhomocysteinaemia in those who carry the mutation. Pregnancy is associated with lower levels of homocysteine, and folic acid supplementation also reduces levels. Whether or not folate supplements can prevent VTE in people with hyperhomocysteinaemia has not been established.

Factor VIII

Factor VIII levels have a dose response relationship with thrombotic risk. Among people with VTE, 20–25% will have factor VIII levels in excess of the 90th centile of the normal population distribution. Blood group (group O subjects have lower levels) and von Willebrand factor levels (VWF is the carrier protein for factor VIII, protecting it from inactivation by aPC) are the major determinants of factor VIII levels. Independent familial transmission of elevated factor VIII levels has not yet been demonstrated.

Fibrinogen
Although abnormal fibrinogens have been described in the context of VTE, thrombotic dysfibrinogenaemias are rare and their relative risk for thrombosis has not been established. High levels of fibrinogen are associated with an increased risk of VTE in the region of four-fold in people with levels in excess of 5 g/l. Specific mutations resulting in hyperfibrinogenaemia have not been identified.

Screening for thrombophilia

As our knowledge of the factors involved in the pathogenesis of thrombosis increases, it is tempting to consider screening for inherited risk factors. Uncertainties remain, however, about the clinical relevance of many of the genotypes and phenotypes described. Some carriers will never develop VTE, and known defects do not account for all cases of VTE, suggesting that additional factors await definition. These two facts mean that assignment of both false positive high risk and false negative low risk is inevitable.

Indiscriminate screening of all patients or of normal populations for thrombophilic defects cannot be recommended at present. Screening should be reserved for those who, on the basis of personal and family history of VTE, are likely to be at increased risk of future VTE, and therefore to benefit from thromboprophylaxis. Those women with a history of three or more consecutive early or late pregnancy losses may also be included. In the obstetric setting, the association between thrombophilic defects and pregnancy complications such as pre-eclampsia, fetal growth restriction and placental abruption may provide a further indication for screening. If screening is to be employed in these situations, it is important that appropriate and effective interventions are identified.

The main benefit in screening is to prevent a first VTE in affected relatives rather than secondary prevention of recurrent VTE. Testing for heritable thrombophilia needs to be undertaken by those in a position to offer family counselling.

Thrombophilia screening should include a coagulation screen (PT, APTT, TT, fibrinogen and FDPs), full blood count, AT and PC activities, PS antigen, lupus anticoagulant test, anticardiolipin antibodies, and determination of factor V and prothrombin 20210A gene status.

Collecting samples for thrombophilia testing is not recommended at the time of an acute VTE event because some tests (AT, PS, PC) are affected by the acute post-thrombotic state and anticoagulants. Furthermore, the finding of an abnormality will not alter the acute management of VTE using standard treatment with heparin and warfarin. Sampling should be delayed until at least one month after completion of an adequate course of anticoagulation, and is best avoided during episodes of acute illness, during pregnancy, and whilst using oral contraceptives or hormone replacement therapy, as all of these situations can influence the circulating levels of pro- and anticoagulant proteins.

Assessment and management of VTE risk

Despite the recent burgeoning of interest and investigation of the pathogenesis of VTE, the clinical relevance of each of the currently identified risk factors and their interactions are still only partially understood. Therefore, the evidence base for the management of patients with VTE and inherited thrombophilia is still weak. In the absence of clinical trial evidence, each individual's risk must be assessed on the basis of common sense and clinical experience. The British Committee for Standards in Haematology (BCSH) has published guidelines for the investigation and management of thrombophilia.[6] Most obstetric units will now have protocols for thromboprophylaxis that take into account all the known risk factors for thrombosis, and the Royal College of Obstetricians and Gynaecologists has produced a guideline addressing the issue of thromboprophylaxis in pregnancy.[9]

Initial estimates of the risk of VTE in pregnancy in women with thrombophilia who were not on anticoagulant therapy were high; however, these data came from observational studies of symptomatic thrombophilic kindreds that overestimated the risk in asymptomatic kindred. Most individuals with a thrombophilic defect will develop VTE only when an additional triggering factor occurs. Different combinations of factors carry different levels of increased risk, and may act additively or synergistically. For example, FVL increases the risk of VTE seven-fold, oral contraceptive pill users have a three-fold increase in risk, but users who are also FVL carriers have a 30-fold increase in VTE risk.

In considering an individual's risk, it is important to consider the absolute level of risk, rather than the relative risk. Starting with a baseline annual risk for age (between one in 10 000 in the under 35s and one in 100 per person per year in the over 75s), the estimated relative risks can be used to calculate the absolute level of risk for any given thrombophilic profile (Table 8.2). Women will differ in their reactions to the same absolute levels of risk, and will therefore make individual choices regarding the acceptability of thromboprophylaxis, alternative contraceptive choices, and the use of hormone replacement therapy.

In general, women may be categorised according to their risk profile (Table 8.3) with respect to future thrombosis. Similar risk assessment

Table 8.2 Estimation of absolute level of VTE risk

Risk factor	Relative risk*	Annual absolute risk		
		<35 years	>50 years	>70 years
Baseline	–	1/10 000	4/10 000	1/100
Pregnancy	x 3	3/10 000	12/10 000	–
Surgery	x 7	7/10 000	28/10 000	7/100
History of VTE	x 8	8/10 000	32/10 000	8/100
OCP	x 3	3/10 000	12/10 000	–
AT deficiency	x 5	5/10 000	20/10 000	5/100
PC deficiency	x 7	7/10 000	28/10 000	7/100
PS deficiency	x 8	8/10 000	32/10 000	8/100
FVL	x 7	7/10 000	28/10 000	7/100
P20210A	x 3	3/10 000	12/10 000	3/100
High factor VIII	x 3	3/10 000	12/10 000	3/100
OCP + FVL	x 30	30/10 000	120/10 000	–

*general estimates of risk taken from various studies

profiles have been developed for women undergoing gynaecological surgery (see Table 7.4, Chapter 7). The estimated level of risk is weighed against the drawbacks or risks of anticoagulation (bleeding and the need for monitoring) to reach an appropriate management strategy. Women in the high risk category should be treated indefinitely with anticoagulants, whereas those in the low risk category should have short-term prophylaxis during periods of heightened risk. The optimal strategy for those in the intermediate category has not been established, and will depend on the individual's valuation of the potential benefits and risks of anticoagulation and conservative approaches.

The management of pregnancy in women with thrombophilia

It is essential that in assessing the risk of thrombosis in pregnancy, both acquired and inherited factors are considered (Table 8.1; see Chapter 7). Although it would seem reasonable that the risk of VTE during pregnancy

Table 8.3 Stratification of patients with respect to future VTE according to the presence of risk factors

Risk profile	Characteristics of patients	Recommended duration of secondary anticoagulant prophylaxis
High	Severe thombophilia* Malignancy Recurrent VTE	Indefinite
Intermediate	Mild thombophilia† Thrombosis in a life-endangering location††	Not well established
Low	Secondary (with transient risk factors§)	Short term (up to 6 months)

*such as antithrombin deficiency, homozygous deficiency of protein C or protein S, homozygous factor V Leiden; †such as heterozygous deficiency of protein C or protein S, heterozygous factor V Leiden or prothrombin gene mutation; ††visceral vein thrombosis, massive pulmonary embolism; §such as surgery, immobilization, pregnancy/puerperium, OCP†

among thrombophilic subjects should be greater, the level of risk has not been firmly established. Most reports are small, suffer from selection bias, and offer incomplete thrombophilia testing. Thus the management of pregnant women with thrombophilic defects remains controversial. To assist decisions, an arbitrary classification of pregnancy-associated VTE risk has been suggested by the British Committee for Standards in Haematology[6] (Table 8.4). It is recommended that these women are assessed, monitored and delivered under the supervision of combined obstetric and haemostasis teams.

All women at risk should be encouraged to wear graduated compression stockings throughout pregnancy and for 6–12 weeks postpartum. Antenatal anticoagulation is achieved using heparin. Most obstetric units now prefer low molecular weight heparin (LMWH), although a specific licence for its use in this area is lacking. Specific therapeutic recommendations for thromboprophylaxis in pregnancy for women with heritable thrombophilia have been made in the current BCSH guidelines[6], and are summarised below (see Table 8.4).

WOMEN WITH SLIGHTLY INCREASED RISK

In general these women do not need antenatal thromboprophylaxis with UFH or LMWH, but should be considered for anticoagulation postdelivery.

Table 8.4 BCSH classification of women at increased risk of pregnancy-associated VTE [6]

Risk category	Description
High risk	Long-term anticoagulants
	AT deficiency
Moderate risk	Previous VTE with or without a thrombophilic defect who are no longer on anticoagulant therapy
	Asymptomatic women who have screen detected heterozygotic PC deficiency or homozygous FVL or PT G20210A mutation, or combination defects
Slightly increased risk	Asymptomatic women who have screen detected heterozygotic PS deficiency, FVL or PT G20210A mutation.
	Previous VTE occurring in the presence of a temporary acquired risk factor that is no longer present, and no identifiable thrombophilic defect

WOMEN AT MODERATE RISK

Fixed prophylactic doses of LMW heparin 4000–5000 anti-Xa units once daily subcutaneously commencing early in pregnancy. Monitoring of anti-Xa activity is not usually necessary, but the platelet count should be checked as for high risk women.

WOMEN AT HIGH RISK

Recommended doses of LMW heparin are higher for this group than usually used for VTE prevention, and thus monitoring and dose adjustment are recommended. A starting dose of LMW heparin 75 anti-Xa units/kg of early pregnancy weight given subcutaneously twice daily throughout pregnancy would be expected to give a peak anti-Xa activity at 3 hours post-injection of 0.35–0.5 units/ml. Peak anti-Xa activity should be checked after the first 4 weeks and 4–6-weekly thereafter. If anti-Xa levels exceed the target range of 0.35–0.5 units/ml, the LMW dose is reduced, and vice versa. Platelet counts should be checked before starting and after 4–8 days of treatment.

Postpartum anticoagulation is required for all women at high or moderately increased risk. This can be achieved using LMWH at a fixed dose as described above, or by changing to warfarin at a sufficient dosage to maintain an INR of 2.0–3.0. Postnatal anticoagulation may be introduced

12 hours after delivery, provided that there is no bleeding, and is continued until discharge, or for 6 weeks in those at higher risk.

Contraception and VTE risk in women with thrombophilia

Oral contraceptives increase the risk of VTE, particularly in the first year of use. Women with thrombophilic defects are at greater risk. The use of the combined oral contraceptive is therefore not recommended for women with a personal history of VTE. Those with a family history in first-degree relatives may also be advised that alternative methods would be preferable. Nevertheless, in women who are asymptomatic, the absolute risks remain low, and the combined oral contraceptive remains the most reliable and acceptable form of contraception for many women, including those with thrombophilic defects. Testing for thrombophilic defects is unlikely to alter these treatment recommendations.

The progestogen content of combined oral contraceptive pills influences the thrombotic risk, with third generation progestogens being associated with a higher risk. In the general population, however, progestogen-only pills do not seem to be associated with an increased risk of VTE. There is no evidence concerning the level of risk in women with thrombophilia, although it is common practice to use progestogen-only pills or impregnated intrauterine devices in women with a personal or family history of VTE.

The arguments for and against screening prior to commencing oral contraceptives include the potential for preventing VTE in high risk subgroups compared with the low population prevalence of heritable defects requiring large numbers to be screened to prevent one event. The issues in screening go far beyond VTE and its sequelae and include psychological, social and cost considerations. As there are no data balancing these aspects, routine screening of all women considering oral contraceptive use is not recommended at present.

Hormone replacement therapy and VTE risk in women with thrombophilia

Although there is evidence to suggest an increased risk of VTE among users of hormone replacement therapy (HRT), there is no reliable information regarding women with thrombophilia. All women starting HRT should be counselled regarding the risk of VTE and should be aware of the signs and symptoms which should lead them to seek further medical advice.

Routine screening of all women for thrombophilic defects prior to commencement of HRT is not warranted. In those women with a personal history of VTE, and in whom the need for HRT is established, consideration may be given to prophylactic treatment with anticoagulants. In those with a family history, and an identified severe thrombophilic defect, this strategy may also be considered. In all cases, the risk of bleeding and the inconvenience of anticoagulant monitoring must be included in the risk–benefit analysis.

For a fuller discussion of the risks of VTE in association with oral contraceptives and hormone replacement therapy, the reader is referred to the review by Rosendaal et al.[10]

Antiphospholipid syndrome

Antiphospholipid syndrome is an acquired thrombophilia, which may be diagnosed when arterial or venous thrombosis or adverse pregnancy outcome occurs in the presence of antiphospholipid antibodies. The syndrome may be a primary disorder, or occur in a secondary setting of rheumatic and connective tissue disorders. The clinical and laboratory criteria for the diagnosis of antiphospholipid syndrome were established by international consensus,[11] and are shown in Table 8.5.

ANTIPHOSPHOLIPID ANTIBODIES

The first of the antiphospholipid antibodies (aPL) to be identified were anticardiolipin antibody and the lupus anticoagulant. It was originally thought that these antibodies reacted with negatively charged phospholipids. It is now known that their true antigenic target is plasma protein bound to an anionic surface, and that reactions with a wide variety of targets are involved in the regulation of coagulation. The most common targets involve B2-glycoprotein and prothrombin, but also include PC, PS, factor XII and tissue-type plasminogen activator, among others. It is thus not difficult to imagine how these antibodies, by interfering with the normal function of regulatory proteins, could produce an imbalance between pro- and anticoagulant systems, with thrombosis as the end result. Nevertheless, a causative role for these antibodies has yet to be firmly established, and an alternative theory speculates that the aPLs are a surrogate marker for a prothrombotic syndrome that has an autoimmune pathogenesis.

Interestingly, aPLs may also occur in relation to the use of some drugs, notably chlorpromazine, and transiently after certain infections. Persistent aPL positivity can occur with chronic infection such as syphilis, hepatitis C and HIV. Furthermore, aPLs may be found incidentally in apparently healthy individuals.

Table 8.5   Criteria for the classification of the antiphospholipid syndrome

Definite antiphospholipid syndrome is considered to be present if at least 1 of the clinical criteria and 1 of the laboratory criteria are met.

Clinical criteria	Vascular thrombosis	One or more episodes of arterial, venous, or small vessel thrombosis in any tissue or organ. Thrombosis must be confirmed by imaging or doppler studies or histopathology, with the exception of superficial venous thrombosis. For histopathological confirmation, thrombosis should be present without significant evidence of inflammation in the vessel wall.
	Pregnancy morbidity	One or more unexplained deaths of a morphologically normal fetus at or beyond the 10th week of gestation, with a normal fetal morphology documented by ultrasound or by direct examination of the fetus. One or more premature births of a morphologically normal neonate at or before the 34th week of gestation because of severe pre-eclampsia or eclampsia, or severe placental insufficiency. Three or more unexplained consecutive spontaneous abortions before the 10th week of gestation, with maternal anatomic or hormonal abnormalities and paternal and maternal chromosomal abnormalities excluded.
Laboratory criteria	Anticardiolipin antibody	IgG and /or IgM isotype in blood, present in medium or high titre, on 2 or more occasions, at least 6 weeks apart, measured by a standardised enzyme-linked immunosorbent assay for B2-glycoprotien I-dependent anticardiolipin antibodies
	Lupus anticoagulant	Present in plasma on 2 or more occasions at least 6 weeks apart, detected according to the guidelines of the International Society on Thrombosis and Haemostasis (Scientific subcommittee on lupus anticoagulants/phospholipid-dependent antibodies), in the following steps: - prolonged phospholipid-dependent coagulation demonstrated on a screening test (APTT, KCT, dilute RVVT, dilute PT, texatarin time) - failure to correct the prolonged coagulation time on the screening test by mixing with normal platelet-poor plasma - shortening or correction of the prolonged coagulation time on the screening test by the addition of excess phospholipids - exclusion of other coagulopathies (FVII inhibitor, heparin)

CLINICAL PRESENTATION OF ANTIPHOSPHOLIPID SYNDROME

Women with antiphospholipid syndrome may present to a wide variety of clinical specialists with venous or arterial thrombosis or obstetric complications. In any situation, it is important to objectively establish the presence of thrombosis as this will determine immediate and long-term management, particularly in women of childbearing age. Clinical features of associated disorders should be sought.

Management of antiphospholipid syndrome

Women with an incidental finding of aPLs have a low level of additional risk for VTE, and therefore antithrombotic therapy is not usually recommended in the absence of a thrombotic event. However, as this group will include women with antiphospholipid syndrome who have not yet experienced their first thrombotic event, it is prudent to recommend short-term prophylaxis in high risk situations such as perioperatively and postpartum.

Consensus on the appropriate management of women with thrombosis and pregnancy complications in the setting of antiphospholipid syndrome is beginning to emerge from clinical studies.

Venous thromboembolism

The initial management of acute VTE is not altered by the diagnosis of antiphospholipid syndrome. Standard therapy with unfractionated or low molecular weight heparin, followed by oral anticoagulation with warfarin, is indicated. A target INR of 2.5 is recommended, although there is still controversy regarding the need for more intensive anticoagulation based on retrospective data suggesting a continuing thrombotic risk with INR values of less than 3.0.

The duration of warfarin therapy is individually assessed, taking into account the presence of any additional remediable risk factors, the severity of the initial event, and the risk of bleeding associated with anticoagulant therapy. Furthermore, with increasing evidence that the thrombosis recurrence rates are particularly high for women with antiphospholipid syndrome, long-term anticoagulation may be beneficial. Current recommendations suggest that treatment for 6 months with a target INR of 2.5 with management of additional risk factors is reasonable. Recurrent thrombosis should be treated with long-term anticoagulation; recurrence while taking warfarin at a target INR of 2.5 should be managed with higher intensity anticoagulation to a target INR of 3.5. The use of oral contraceptives and HRT are best avoided in women with aPLs and thrombosis, but may be considered in women on warfarin therapy.

Arterial thrombosis

There is a high risk of recurrence with the likelihood of permanent disability or death as the result of stroke. Therefore cerebral infarction in women with antiphospholipid syndrome should be managed with long-term anticoagulation with warfarin at a target INR of 2.5. The benefit of the addition of aspirin has not yet been established, but the risk of haemorrhage is increased.

Extracerebral arterial thromboembolism is also an indication for long-term anticoagulation with warfarin. In all cases, attention should be given to the control of additional risk factors.

Thrombocytopenia

When thrombocytopenia is the only manifestation of antiphospholipid syndrome, management is essentially similar to that recommended for women with idiopathic thrombocytopenic purpura (ITP). The treatment options will include steroid, immunoglobulin and splenectomy. In situations where there is thrombocytopenia and thrombosis, anticoagulant therapy will be associated with a greater bleeding risk. Where the thrombocytopenia is modest (in the region of $50 \times 10^9/l$) and thrombosis is the principal manifestation, anticoagulation should still be considered.

Pregnancy failure

Antiphospholipid antibodies are present in only 2% of women with a low risk obstetric history compared with 15% of women with recurrent miscarriage, in whom the live birth rate in untreated pregnancies may be as low as 10%.[12] The underlying mechanisms that cause pregnancy morbidity in antiphospholipid syndrome are thought to be inhibition of trophoblastic function and differentiation in early pregnancy, and later on, thrombosis of the uteroplacental vasculature.[12]

A variety of interventions have been used to try to improve pregnancy outcomes in women with antiphospholipid syndrome. Available data are limited by small numbers of women studied, varying eligibility criteria and treatment protocols, and the lack of laboratory standardisation of aPL assays. A 2002 systematic review of the evidence for potential therapies included ten studies that met their inclusion criteria.[13] Three trials of aspirin alone showed no significant reduction in pregnancy loss; two trials showed that heparin combined with aspirin significantly reduced pregnancy loss when compared with aspirin alone; prednisolone and aspirin resulted in an increase in prematurity but no significant reduction in pregnancy loss. There is no evidence that steroids improve the live birth rate and their use is associated with significant maternal and fetal morbidity.[12] However, the live birth rate is improved (up to 70%) when combination therapy of aspirin plus heparin is prescribed.[12]

It is therefore recommended that women with a history of recurrent miscarriage associated with persistent aPLs should be treated with aspirin 75 mg/day as soon as the pregnancy test becomes positive, and low dose heparin commenced when fetal heart activity is seen on ultrasound. Unfractionated heparin 5000 units subcutaneously twice daily was the highest dose administered in any study; LMWH has not been shown in any clinical trial to be equivalent or better, but is increasingly used.

The optimal duration of therapy with aspirin and heparin has not been established, but prolonged use of heparin is not recommended because of the risk of osteopenia. For women with a history of early pregnancy events, stopping at 34 weeks may be reasonable, while those with late pregnancy events will require treatment to be continued to term. Those women with a history of thrombosis should have postpartum thromboprophylaxis. Women receiving heparin and aspirin should have a platelet count checked weekly for the first three weeks and 4–6 weekly thereafter.

Although treatment with aspirin plus heparin significantly improves the live birth rate, these pregnancies remain at high risk of complications including recurrent miscarriage, pre-eclampsia, fetal growth restriction and preterm birth, and close antenatal surveillance is essential.[11] Regular obstetric assessment including Doppler ultrasound is recommended to detect complications at an early stage, and ready availability of a suitable neonatal unit is necessary.

Summary

Venous thromboembolism is a common cause of morbidity and mortality and has been implicated in the pathophysiology of a number of obstetric complications. VTE is a multifactorial disease involving the interaction of genetic and environmental factors. However, our knowledge regarding the clinical relevance of all of the possible risk factors remains incomplete. The presence and interactions of transient or persistent risk factors for VTE, as well as their different strengths in triggering thrombosis must be taken into account for a valid approach to issues in screening and in making decisions about the use of primary and secondary prophylaxis of VTE with anticoagulant drugs.

Key points

- Venous thromboembolism (VTE) is a common cause of morbidity and mortality in obstetric and gynaecological practice.
- Thrombosis has been implicated in the pathophysiology of a number of obstetric complications.
- VTE is a multifactorial disease involving the interaction of genetic and environmental factors.
- Thrombophilia refers to situations associated with increased risk of VTE characterised by hypercoaguability.
- The most common genetic factors are deficiencies of the naturally occurring anticoagulants AT, PC and PS, and the FVL and prothrombin G20210A mutations.
- Screening for thrombophilia should be reserved for those with a family history of VTE, a personal history of unexplained or unusual VTE, recurrent early pregnancy loss, fetal growth restriction or placental abruption.
- Assessment of transient or persistent risk factors for VTE is necessary to establish the need for primary or secondary VTE prophylaxis and in making choices about oral contraceptives or hormone replacement therapy.
- Discussion of individual risk should be conducted in terms of the absolute levels of risk.
- Antiphospholipid syndrome is an acquired thrombophilia characterised by thrombosis or recurrent pregnancy loss in association with antiphospholipid antibodies.
- Improved pregnancy outcomes in women with antiphospholipid syndrome can be achieved with the use of aspirin and low-dose heparin.

References

1 Bertina RM. Molecular Risk Factors for Thrombosis. *Thromb Haemost* 1999;82(2):601–9.

2 McColl MD, Walker ID, Greer IA. The role of inherited thrombophilia in venous thromboembolism associated with pregnancy. *Br J Obstet Gynaecol* 1999;106:756–66.

3 Rosendaal FR. Risk Factors for Venous Thrombotic Disease. *Thromb Haemost* 1999;82(2):610–19.

4 Greaves M, Cohen H, Machin SJ, Mackie I. Guidelines on the investigation and management of the antiphospholipid syndrome. *Br J Haematol* 2000;109:704–15.

5 Martinelli I. Risk factors in venous thromboembolism. *Thromb Haemost* 2001;86:395–403.

6 Walker ID, Greaves M, Preston FE, for the Haemostasis and Thrombosis Task Force of the British Committee for Standards in Haematology. Guideline: Investigation and Management of Heritable Thrombophilia. *Br J Haematol* 2001;114:512–28.

7 De Stefano V, Rossi E, Paciaroni K, Leone G. Screening for inherited thrombophilia: indications and therapeutic implications. *Haematologica* 2002;87(10):1095–1108.

8 Schafer AI, Levine MN, Konkle BA, Kearon C. Thrombotic disorders: diagnosis and treatment. *Hematology (Am Soc Hematol Educ Program)* 2003;520–39.

9 Royal College of Obstetricians and Gynaecologists. *Thromboprophylaxis during pregnancy, labour and after delivery*. Guideline No. 37. London: RCOG; 2004.

10 Rosendaal FR, Helmerhorst FM, Vandenbroucke JP. Oral contraceptives, hormone replacement therapy and thrombosis. *Thromb Haemost* 2001;86:112–23.

11 Wilson WA, Gharavi AE, Koike T, *et al*. International Consensus Statement on preliminary classification criteria for definite antiphospholipid syndrome. Report of an International Workshop. *Arthritis Rheum* 1999;42(7):1309–11.

12 Royal College of Obstetricians and Gynaecologists. *The investigation and treatment of couples with recurrent miscarriage. Guideline No. 17*. London: RCOG; 2003.

13 Empson M, Lassere M, Craig JC, Scott JR. Recurrent pregnancy loss with antiphospholipid antibody: a systematic review of therapeutic trials. *Obstet Gynaecol* 2002;99:135–44.

Index

ablation 85
activated partial prothrombin time
    (APTT) 66–7, 101
air travel 95
amniotic fluid embolism 63
anaemia 80
anaphylaxis 92, 93
antenatal diagnosis/screening
    fetus 18–19, 21, 23, 36
    mother 45, 100, 115
antepartum haemorrhage 43, 44–8, 62–3
    treatment 46, 48, 50–4
antibiotics 50
anticardiolipin antibodies 121, 122
anticoagulants
    at parturition 103–4
    natural 8–10
        deficiencies 98, 112–13
        DIC 60, 63–4, 67–8, 69–70
    thromboprophylaxis 92–4, 96–9,
        118–20
    treatment of acute VTE 101–3, 123
antiphospholipid syndrome 121–5
antishock garments 52
antithrombin
    deficiency 98, 112, 113
    DIC 60, 63–4, 67–8, 69
    haemostasis 8–9
anti-Xa 96, 101, 102
aPC see protein C, activated
aprotinin 10
APTT (activated partial prothrombin
    time) 66–7, 101
arterial embolisation 55
arterial thrombosis 124
aspirin 93–4, 97, 124–5
autoimmune thrombocytopenia 5, 29–30

balloon catheters 52, 85

beta human chorionic gonadotrophin
    (βhCG) 44
B-Lynch technique 52
breastfeeding 20, 94, 96

caesarean section
    bleeding disorders 21, 22
    obstetric haemorrhage 46, 48
    thrombocytopenia 30, 34
    VTE 90–1, 96, 103–4
carboprost 49
cardiotocography 48
cerebrovascular accidents 124
cervix 45
chlorpromazine 121
chorionic villus sampling 18–19
Christmas disease see haemophilia carriers
coagulation system 1, 6–10, 66
    see also individual factors
colloids 51
computed tomography (CT) 100
contraceptives
    LNG-IUS 83–4
    oral 9, 77, 81–2, 104–5, 120
cord blood 21
cryoprecipitate 22
crystalloids 51

dalteparin see low-molecular-weight
    heparin
danazol 83
DDAVP (desmopressin) 20, 22, 23, 82–3
D-dimer 63, 67, 100–1
deep vein thrombosis (DVT)
    diagnosis 99–100
    long-term effects 90
    postoperative 91, 93, 94–5, 101
    in pregnancy 92, 94, 101
desmopressin (DDAVP) 20, 22, 23, 82–3
dextran 93
digital vaginal examination 45
dilutional coagulopathy 51, 53
disseminated intravascular coagulation
    (DIC)
    acute 62–3, 65–6
    chronic 61, 62, 63–5, 66, 69
    diagnosis 65–8
    key points 70
    management 28–9, 65, 68–70